THE END OF STRESS

"With stress emerging as a primary contributor to eroding employee engagement, health, well-being, productivity, and overall performance, companies that can teach their workforces how to manage stress better than their rivals will achieve a significant competitive advantage. What makes *The End of Stress* so compelling is that it converts decades of research, science, and evidence-based practices into a practical, pragmatic program that real people can use to dramatically transform their performance, their success, and their lives. A must-read for anyone interested in improving human performance—their own or others'."

—**Eric Severson**, Global Vice President
for Human Resources, Gap Inc.

"There is no one better qualified than Don Joseph Goewey to offer you a solution to stress that paves the way to a powerful brain to lift your life even higher than where you currently stand. Take my word for it, this book will enable you to attain that goal."

—**Gerald G. Jampolsky, MD**, author of
Love Is Letting Go of Fear and coauthor of *A Mini Course for Life*

"As an epidemiologist, I can attest that nearly every ailment we suffer from today is caused, triggered, or exacerbated by stress. We're overeating, drinking, and smoking because we're stressed. We're suffering from stress-induced illnesses—from acute disorders like headaches, digestive disorders, and sleep disorders to more serious problems like heart attacks, cancer, and premature aging. Stress also strains our relationships with our family, coworkers, and friends. And if all this isn't bad enough, stress hormones debilitate the higher brain function that enables you to excel in your career. In the midst of all this bad news is the good news that Don Joseph Goewey brings, which is this: You can literally rewire your brain to be stress-resistant by making a specific shift in mind-set. The process of change is simpler than you might imagine, and results accrue faster than you might think. Want to improve your health, transform a failing relationship, and reach greater heights in your career? Read *The End of Stress*."

—**Barbara Wexler**, epidemiologist, medical writer,
and author of *Reducing Stress*

"If your life is hard because of STRESS . . . this book is for you! Don Joseph Goewey creates a clear, simple, calming pathway that will move you from chaos to peace of mind. Don does a beautiful job of not only explaining why and how we experience stress but gives us tools, stories, and techniques for creating a lifelong practice that attains that powerful and empowering state of being called stress-free."

—**Jim Horan**, president of
The One Page Business Plan Company
and author of *The One Page Business Plan*

THE
END
OF
STRESS

THE
END
OF
STRESS

FOUR STEPS TO REWIRE YOUR BRAIN

DON JOSEPH GOEWEY

ATRIA PAPERBACK
New York London Toronto Sydney New Delhi

BEYOND WORDS
Hillsboro, Oregon

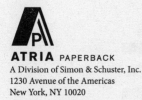

ATRIA PAPERBACK
A Division of Simon & Schuster, Inc.
1230 Avenue of the Americas
New York, NY 10020

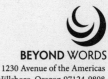

BEYOND WORDS
1230 Avenue of the Americas
Hillsboro, Oregon 97124-9808
503-531-8700 / 503-531-8773 fax
www.beyondword.com

This publication contains the opinions and ideas of its author. It is intended to provide helpful and informative material on the subjects addressed in the publication. It is sold with the understanding that the author and publisher are not engaged in rendering medical, health, or any other kind of personal professional services in the book. The reader should consult his or her medical, health, or other competent professional before adopting any of the suggestions in this book or drawing inferences from it. The author and publisher specifically disclaim all responsibility for any liability, loss, or risk, personal or otherwise, that is incurred as a consequence, directly or indirectly, of the use and application of any of the contents of this book.

Managing editor: Lindsay S. Brown
Editors: Sarah Heilman, Emily Han
Copyeditor: Meadowlark Publishing Services
Proofreader: Linda M. Meyer
Design: Devon Smith
Composition: William H. Brunson Typography Services

First Atria Paperback/Beyond Words trade paperback edition September 2014

For more information about special discounts for bulk purchases, please contact Simon & Schuster Special Sales at 1-866-506-1949 or business@simonandschuster.com.

The Simon & Schuster Speakers Bureau can bring authors to your live event. For more information or to book an event, contact the Simon & Schuster Speakers Bureau at 1-866-248-3049 or visit our website at www.simonspeakers.com.

Manufactured in the United States of America

10 9 8 7 6 5 4 3 2

Library of Congress Cataloging-in-Publication Data

Goewey, Don Joseph.
    The end of stress : four steps to rewire your brain / Don Joseph Goewey.
        pages   cm
    1. Stress (Psychology).   2. Anxiety.   3. Stress management.   4. Neuroplasticity.   I. Title.
    BF575.S75G577 2014
    155.9'042—dc23
                                                                    2014011055

ISBN 978-1-58270-491-3
ISBN 978-1-4767-7145-8 (eBook)

The corporate mission of Beyond Words Publishing, Inc.: *Inspire to Integrity*

CONTENTS

Deserted beach,
footsteps in the sand
erased by rain—
this anguish comes from nowhere,
and its feet do not yet touch the Earth.

Suddenly I hear a far-off whisper
of the gentle winds of Spring,
and the anguish is gone.

—Thich Nhat Hanh

"Unclasp" from *Call Me by My True Names:*
The Collected Poems of Thich Nhat Hanh

Foreword

Nearly twenty-five years ago, Don Goewey walked into my office on the docks of Tiburon and sat in a chair across from me by the window that overlooked San Francisco Bay. He had come to interview for the chief executive position at the International Center for Attitudinal Healing (ICAH),* the agency that I'd cofounded more than a decade before. He had great credentials. He'd worked as an executive at my alma mater, Stanford Medical School, and before that had been an associate of Carl Rogers. Of course, I had no idea at the time that I was meeting a person I would someday call my *mensch*. If you don't know what *mensch* means, it's a Yiddish word describing a person to admire and emulate. It's someone of noble character. But Don was not only to become dear to my heart; he would become a partner to me in bringing the agency's psychological approach to some of the world's toughest venues, from war zones, prisons, and poor communities to the stress-plagued environment of corporate America.

---

* ICAH is the International Center for Attitudinal Healing; the center was renamed Attitudinal Healing International in 2010.

At that time, ICAH was a kind of proving ground for an emerging school of psychology I'd initiated based on the power of attitude. The approach defined health as inner peace, and healing as letting go of fear. It asserted that it isn't people or events that cause us distress, but rather our own thoughts, feelings, and attitudes toward people and events. The aim of the programs the center pioneered was to help people transcend the anxiety, stress, and depression of catastrophic situations by making the fundamental shift in attitude from fear to peace. In facing adversity, it's common to relate to the stress-provoking images that a fearful mind-set perceives, not as a choice, but as reality.

Conversely, most people relate to peace (if they relate to it at all) as a complacent, demotivated state of mind that's emphasized once a year on holiday cards and then set aside. Peace is not generally regarded as the pinnacle of personal power, and fear is not seen as the loss of that power. Thousands of people who came to the center for support would beg to differ. Nearly all of them made the shift from fear to peace in dealing with ordinary life crises, from divorce or losing a job in a bad economy to what might seem to be insurmountable challenges, such as cancer, AIDS, paralysis, or the loss of a loved one. These clients would tell you that the attitudinal shift from fear to peace is no small thing. It generates a change in the way you see and relate to life that can change everything. That's because attitude is the psychological force that can move you from feeling overwhelmed by circumstances to a way of being that makes you larger than circumstances. It's the last of human freedoms, to quote Viktor Frankl, bestowing the power to choose your own experience inside, regardless of what's happening outside.[1] Master the power of attitude and you'll live a powerful life. The center was so successful in demonstrating the capacity of ordinary people to make this extraordinary shift that *60 Minutes* reported on it, and a documentary film about the center's children's program won a Peabody Award.

In the years since I founded the center, neuroscience has established that a peaceful mind is also the key to unlocking the brain's full potential. In the last decade, medical science has established that our mental state even determines how healthy our bodies will be, right down to the molecular level of our cells and chromosomes.

So, getting back to Don: For the twelve years that he directed the center, he ventured into places of extreme fear and despair and helped people facilitate the shift to peace. When he wasn't doing that, he was immersed in the neuroscience that was beginning to explain how this shift in attitude literally produced positive changes in the brain. Eventually, Don accepted a challenge to take what he was learning about the brain and integrate it with everything he knew from his work with people in order to build a model that could end stress. It took nearly six years, but Don succeeded in ways no one else has, as thousands of people who have been touched by this work would attest. Here is one example, from an intensive care nurse:

> This course has changed my life! That sounds dramatic, but in the past few days, my whole perspective and approach have been dramatically different. I am making a conscious effort to shift my attitude and approach to all that I do. So far, it has given me such peace and hope. It is really a healing and inspiring course. I have heard many different people's approaches to stress management and actualization of total wellness, but none of them reached me the way this has.

Here is another example from an executive at a multinational corporation:

> This course has the ability to engage us all in the formation of our best selves, and to that end I hope this course flourishes in all venues.

This is the opportunity for change that Don's new book extends to you.

Sometimes when people read a book that inspires personal transformation, they might think the author is someone who managed to avoid the pain or struggle they're attempting to overcome. This is rarely the case and is definitely not the case with Don. He had to overcome a painful childhood with a father who abandoned him and a stepfather who was abusive. By Don's own account, for years he struggled with anger, fear, and shame until life forced him to face himself. The catalyst was losing his job and being diagnosed with a brain tumor, all in the same week. If that wasn't bad enough, he was also married with four small children, and the marriage was crumbling.

When the stress and fear he felt over this set of circumstances finally reached the point of being unbearable, Don somehow managed to open his heart enough to allow grace to step into this dark moment and turn on a light. Don found himself asking which was worse: the circumstances he faced, or how terrified and immobilized he'd become? That question led to Don realizing how much and how long he'd lived with stress and anger. He made the decision right then and there to walk in the opposite direction, toward the light at the end of the tunnel, no matter what happened next. He committed himself to seeing life through the eyes of peace. It produced a sea change in him, a sea change we are all capable of making. Certainly, since his transforming moment of grace, Don's anger and fear have raised their heads, but not without him shifting away from them. He is focused on and committed to working through any negative pattern that interferes with the empowering experience of peace. He owns his mistakes and forgives them, and because of that, he's developed an empathic heart that steers him away from judging other people.

Don has put it all in this book—his experience, his knowledge, and his heart. In my opinion, there is no one better qualified to offer you a solution to stress that can pave the way to a powerful brain to lift your life even higher. Take my word for it: you are in very good hands.

—Gerald G. Jampolsky, MD, author of *Love Is Letting Go of Fear* and coauthor of *A Mini Course for Life*

Introduction:
The Bad News and the
Exceedingly Good News

This book is about a solution to stress, which is essentially the neuroscience of success or how to locate the mental zone that enables higher-brain networks to perform optimally. When these networks wire and fire together, humming away happily at the brain speed of a hundred million computer instructions per second,[1] you excel at every level of life, from career to family, from physical and emotional well-being to a lower golf score. It's a brain generating the analytic and creative intelligence to achieve your goals, along with the emotional and social intelligence to instill joy in your work, peace in your life, and harmony in your relationships. It's also the key to health and longevity. All of these positive outcomes are what nature intended when it evolved the higher brain. The bad news is that stress debilitates, erodes, and even damages higher-brain networks, inhibiting you from living and succeeding fully. The good news is there is now a solution to stress that not only repairs the damage stress causes but also generates the neurological conditions that stimulate the growth of new connections within the higher brain, expanding brain capacity. As these networks integrate, they make you a more fully functioning whole, able to reach even greater heights.

I want to start by reviewing the really bad news about stress to underline its impact, and then unveil for you the profoundly good news about the solution to stress that builds a powerful brain. To begin with, stress reactions produce stress hormones, and stress hormones disable the higher brain's executive functions that allow you to first make a plan and then manage it through to completion. Stress hormones shrink other networks, as well, and break the connections between them, rendering you incapable of sustaining peak performance or generating the creative insight that leads to innovation. These hormones lock you into fight, flight, or freeze mode and switch your emotional set point to negative, predisposing you to feeling anxiety, anger, paranoia, and depression. They impair the immune system, wreak havoc on the cardiovascular system, damage chromosomes, kill brain cells, and, if left unchecked, will eventually kill you.

If you add up all the deaths caused by stress-related illnesses—heart disease, strokes, cancer, immunodeficiency, diabetes, and premature aging, to name a few—you have the number-one cause of death in America today. Stress may even be addictive. During an extreme stress response, the body naturally produces endogenous opioid peptides that mimic the effects of morphine and heroin.[2] In some experiments, severely stressed lab animals exhibited withdrawal symptoms when researchers stopped stressing them, suggesting chemical dependency.[3] It's arguable that life in the fast lane of modern culture is turning us into "stressaholics."

The head of a public relations firm once told me that it took him twenty years to finally realize that what people want most is health, wealth, and love. I think he's right. We want to avoid heart attacks, strokes, and cancer. We want to do well in our careers and make good money. And we want to be happy and enjoy our family and friends. Stress inhibits brain networks (aka neural networks) designed to secure these positive outcomes.

But don't stress about it. The good news about stress is *really good*. There's a solution to the problem that restores your brain so it can fulfill its mission, which is enabling you to flourish at every level of life that matters to you. This book facilitates that solution, and what makes this really good news even better is that the path to a solution is quite simple. It involves using a set of tools that nearly anyone can learn and apply and which, when integrated into your daily life, add virtually nothing to your to-do list. In fact, quieting stress reactions and amplifying higher-brain function are all about actualizing a *to-be* list.

Nearly all the tools and processes you are going to learn are proven, either through research or clinical experience. This book comes out of my years of work, first as the director of the International Center for Attitudinal Healing (ICAH), an agency that pioneered a cutting-edge approach to overcoming catastrophic life events, and more recently as managing partner of ProAttitude, a human performance firm consulting with corporations to alleviate work stress.

At ICAH, we worked in some of the most stressful places on the planet: on cancer and AIDS wards with people facing death, in grief groups with parents who had lost children, at prisons with men serving life sentences, and in refugee camps with people suffering from posttraumatic stress disorders inflicted by the genocidal war in Bosnia. The agency's approach facilitated a shift in attitude aimed at alleviating the fear and stress endemic in these desperate situations, and the results ICAH achieved earned it an international reputation.

My focus on work stress began one day when I was still at ICAH. That day, Larry Stupski, one of the great business minds in recent times, came to see me. Larry and Chuck Schwab raised Charles Schwab & Company to the height it eventually reached. Larry had survived a nearly fatal heart attack caused by years of extreme stress, and he came to me to propose funding a kind of think tank to morph the agency's approach into a model that could end work stress as we know it. At the time it seemed implausible to me, but this was a man of great vision and enormous intellect, and he was confident this goal could be achieved.

Soon thereafter, we were joined by Bonny Meyer, another business visionary. Bonny was cofounder of Silver Oak Cellars, which helped establish the Napa Valley as one of the great wine-producing regions of the world. She, too, was confident we could create a solution to stress. So I accepted the challenge, assembled a team of experts, and went to work on the problem. Our timing was fortunate, coinciding with a string of major breakthroughs in research on stress and the brain.

After six years of hard work, we emerged with a solution to stress that went far beyond conventional stress management. We then ventured out into the real world and applied this new approach in large, high-pressure organizations, achieving impressive results. The average overall rating the course has achieved so far is 4.8 out of 5.0 on the Likert scale, which is rarely achieved in any training.* This indicates a high level of assimilation that predicts a change in company culture, which is exactly what we've seen happen. More than 90 percent of participants experienced a change in their level of stress, which they expected would continue to decline as they practiced what they learned. In addition, more than three out of four participants experienced improvement in creative problem solving, well-being, and their work and family relationships. Make no mistake: you can, too.

In chapter 1, I outline for you the high points of what we discovered about the problem, its solution, and the model we built that paves the way to ending stress. It provides a way to understand the neurology and genetics behind stress, and the breakthroughs in research that define the solution.

How to Use This Book

If you give this book the opportunity to guide you in this new direction, you will emerge from this experience with a brain that sustains you at the top of your game, delivering your best day, every day. This book offers a clear path to the health, wealth, and love we all want. Recently, a journalist writing an article on stress for a national magazine asked me, "What's the secret to changing from 'easily stressed' to 'rarely stressed'?" There is no secret. It's a matter of practicing, over a six- to eight-week period, simple tools and processes that build the specific mind-set that transcends stress. As you do, your brain begins to change in ways that enable you to flourish. And it's not as difficult or as taxing as you might think. Changing a brain wired for a frustrating life of stress has to do with learning and then practicing a to-be list, which defines nothing more and nothing less than how you want to be as you do whatever you have to do. Practice it every day and your brain's autopilot gradually switches from one wired for stress to one that runs an algorithm of emotional calm and mental clarity, even when under siege. The reward is higher-brain networks functioning at optimum levels to increase the odds you will succeed at what matters most to you.

The End of Stress is designed to guide you through that change. This book is not meant to be read quickly from cover to cover in a few days. Rather, it is a guided process that moves you along gradually, like a training seminar. The chapters provide the context and the scientific basis for the tools described. The step-by-step process for using each of the tools is presented at the end of the chapter. Some tools are linked to an audio file you can download that guides you through the process of using that tool.

At the end of each chapter I have also included a section called Your Practice This Week, where I assign practices for you to follow. After reading this section, don't jump to the next chapter. Instead, work with the tools I've assigned for a few days—I recommend five days to a week—before reading the next section. As you perform your practice, review the chapter you just read to remind yourself of why the practice is important. Practicing consistently achieves the greatest change in brain function. The more you use the tools, the easier it gets. Eventually you will reach the point where you can bust a burgeoning stress reaction at the point of inception.

A Four-Step Process

This book guides you through a four-step process. These steps build the awareness that opens the door to choice and defines the choices that shift your experience from stress to peace. They then help you master the tools and processes, not only to sustain the shift but to expand upon it so you can reach your highest potential.

Step 1: Building Awareness—The Insight That Ends Stress as You Know It

> In the first phase you will begin to bring your stress pattern into greater awareness to slow down stress reactions and empower the choice for peace.

Step 2: Getting to Choice—The Mind-Set That Transforms Your Brain

> In the second phase, you will learn and then practice a specific set of principles leading to choices that facilitate positive brain change.

Step 3: Expanding Beyond Stress—Keys to Tapping Your Brain's Full Potential

> By the third phase, you're becoming skillful at transcending stress at the point of inception. In the absence of toxic stress hor-

mones, the higher brain begins to heal and expand, enabling you to actualize more of your brain's innate potential.

Step 4: Sustaining It—Every Day in Every Way
The End of Stress exposes you to a number of proven processes and tools. Each one facilitates the same change of becoming stress free. You may prefer some of the tools over others. In the final step you take using this book, you'll consolidate the tools that worked best for you into an individual practice for moving forward on your own.

QR Tags and the Book's Website for Downloading Course Materials

You will find multimedia QR tags throughout most of the book, usually at the end of the chapters. QR tags are two-dimensional bar codes that create an automatic link to specific audio files that guide you in using a tool from a particular chapter. On page 215, you will find a list of all the audio files in one place and the link to the website where they are collected. There is also a QR tag at the back of the book to sign-up for my newsletter for the latest breakthroughs in neuroscience and new stress-busting tools. You can use your smartphone to download one of many free apps to scan the QR tags, or you can type the link address into any internet browser.

You can also download the audio files, as well as worksheets, tools, and other materials related to this book at theendofstress book.com.

1

A Brain Wired for Stress and the Attitude That Rewires It

The American Psychological Association (APA) annually conducts a survey called Stress in America that is considered our best stress barometer. In its most recent survey, the APA concluded that the data "portrays a picture of high stress and ineffective coping mechanisms that appear to be ingrained in our culture, perpetuating unhealthy lifestyles and behaviors for future generations."[1] The goal of this book is bold but achievable; it's to break that chain by providing a clear path for resolving this crisis once and for all, beginning with you.

As we set out on this journey toward becoming stress free, let me be perfectly clear about one thing: stress is serious. It's life-threatening serious. To quote Carol Shively from the *National Geographic* documentary *Killer Stress*, "It's not something that maybe someday you should do something about. You need to attend to it today."[2] Today, before you end up on a gurney in the emergency room with doctors and nurses treating your heart attack or stroke. The tools and processes in this book greatly increase the odds of you avoiding serious health crises.

I want to give you some sense of what my think tank and I discovered about the seriousness of stress, its definitive solution,

1

and the model that paves the way to all the positive outcomes I just mentioned.

During our research, the first thing we learned was that there are two major brain systems that determine the degree to which you will actualize the brain power to succeed at life.

The first system is called the higher brain. Its proper name is the prefrontal cortex, and much of what we define as human intelligence is generated in this part of the brain. The higher brain invented art, music, science, agriculture, engineering, commerce, government, and lots of other things. It is also where the brain's chief executive has its office, performing the executive functions that produce the plans and strategies that achieve goals. Executive functions draw on all the higher-order cognitive skills that question perceptions, analyze facts, adapt to change, and integrate information—delineating and priori-tizing the logistics that move plans forward. Executive functions also take the creative insight generated by the right brain and translate it into practical innovation.

The higher brain is also the place where the "better angels" of your nature reside, enabling you to sustain constructive, positive relationships and to think beyond a limited self-interest for the greater good. In *Mindsight*, neuropsychiatrist Daniel Siegel locates these angels in the middle portion of the prefrontal area, where they coordinate an astonishing number of essential skills to pro-duce social intelligence. These angels attune you to other people, balance your emotions, enable you to be flexible in your responses, soothe your fear, and generate your capacity for empathy, insight, and intuition.[3]

The higher brain is so much more than what I've described here. It's arguably evolution's greatest single achievement—borne out in the multiple intelligences and aptitudes the cortex produces, and evident in the ancient and modern wonders of the world that it has created. The evolutionary process that built the higher brain bordered on the miraculous. The swiftness at which it developed is unparalleled in the evolutionary record.[4] It was like the waving of a wand.

When this highly evolved brain is functioning optimally, every day can be amazing, filled with enthusiasm, social intelligence, and the joy of excelling. In my last book, *Mystic Cool*, I attempted to describe one of those amazing days when your higher brain flows with the ordinary genius that makes you believe you can accomplish anything. I wrote:

> From time to time, each of us has experienced the glory of the ordinary genius [the higher brain generates] when attempting to accomplish something meaningful that stretches our abilities. The usual storm of demands, pressures, and doubts may have been present at the outset, but by subtle twists and turns, you managed to slip past the storm and locate the eye, where the pressure to produce became the challenge to excel. As you settled in, an effortless flow of intelligence took over, sweeping you along in its inevitable current. Your mind became clear and worked with precision. Time stood still. You felt exhilarated and were able to channel, focus, and conserve your enthusiasm, maintaining a high level of energy. Gradually you began to exhibit surprising mastery over the task at hand, preserving a vision of the whole even as you attended to details. Pieces fell effortlessly into place, as if the dots were connecting themselves. Your sense of the whole was expanded as wider possibilities emerged. Working in this way did not feel like work at all. Rather, it became a rewarding labor of love.[5]

This is the experience the ancient Greeks defined as joy, and it depends entirely on a fully functioning higher brain. Mihaly Csikszentmihalyi, the father of Positive Psychology, said, "Once we have tasted this joy, we will redouble our efforts to taste it again. This is the way the self grows."[6] It's also the way higher-brain network integrates and expands.

The second system is the lower or primitive brain, which actually inhibits your potential for success. The lower brain is where the stress response system resides, and the stress response system, as well as much of the primitive brain, is governed by the brain's fear center, the amygdala. The amygdala plays a substantial role in negative mental states such as distress, aggression, anxiety, depression, and all those emotions that fall under the heading of fight, flight, or freeze.

The amygdala cannot distinguish a real and present danger from something you misperceive as a threat. Its intelligence is reactive, not analytic. It invites the higher brain to weigh in on a potentially threatening situation only if it's a new experience.[7] When your nervous system senses any kind of a threat, a signal is sent to the thalamus (a kind of neurological switchboard) and then relayed to the amygdala to activate an aggressive or defensive reaction. The sequence from threat to fear response happens in a knee-jerk fashion at lightning speed and occurs outside of conscious awareness. The amygdala is a survival system, which means it doesn't take chances. Its motto is "He who hesitates is dead." Thus, it's programmed to shoot first and ask questions later. When there is a real and present danger, such as a coiled rattlesnake on the path, the speed of the amygdala works to increase the odds of living another day.

But most humans no longer live in the wilderness, where lightning reactions are critical to survival. We function within the safety of civilized social settings where fight, flight, or freeze gets us into trouble. The fear-based amygdala makes us delusional by reading threats into situations that aren't actually there. This tendency is the result of "contextual fear conditioning."

Joseph LeDoux of New York University described contextual fear conditioning in his groundbreaking book *The Emotional Brain.* He states that if you place a rat in a box and shock it a number of times while simultaneously sounding a tone, the rat will become fear-conditioned to that tone; from then on, the tone will trigger a fear reaction. But the rat will also become fear-conditioned to the box, which represents the context in which the shock trauma occurred. Simply placing the rat back in the box will set off a stress reaction, even in the absence of the tone.[8]

This research illustrates how during intense stress, the amygdala stores all sorts of information about what is happening around us. In fact, all of our past traumas are stored in an aspect of the brain commonly referred to as emotional memory. Emotional memory is the core problem in the painful and sometimes insane posttraumatic stress reactions of war veterans. When the amygdala finds that one or more of these stored elements matches something in a present situation, it can set off a flashback or memory that triggers fight, flight, or freeze. The amygdala is playing a kind of name-that-tune game, and it is happening continually. The amygdala assigns meaning to what's currently going on outside based on telltale features of traumatic memories stored on the inside, and then guides our emotional behavior accordingly. For example, we can actually dislike, fear, or even attack someone because the amygdala associates a trait in that person with someone who hurt us in the past.

I was once condescending and dismissive toward a consultant who was presenting critical information during an important business meeting. I had just met this woman and had no personal history with her. I am not given to being caustic or rude with people, so my behavior made no sense. The woman tried to make the best of an unpleasant situation, but she didn't get far. It was clear to everyone, including her, that I didn't like her or trust what she had to say. It wasn't until much later, when I was alone, that it suddenly dawned on me that this woman's manner and appearance resembled someone who had caused me a great deal of pain years before. This was the stimulus that drove my behavior in the meeting. Emotional memory activated me to such a degree that I couldn't remember much of what the consultant had said. The emotional brain had me too focused on disliking this woman to be able to hear her.

When the amygdala associates something in the present situation with an upset stored in emotional memory, things can get even uglier, causing us to react with the same fury that might have been relevant to the original threat but is completely inappropriate in the current situation. It's the past usurping the present, which is why psychologists say you're rarely upset for the reason you think. If your higher brain recognizes the negative pattern, it will step in to keep emotional reactions under control. But this takes a significant mental effort that comes at the expense of being intelligent about and attentive to what's happening at present. You're basically locked into trying to control the emotional negativity going on inside of you instead of managing what's happening around you. You're blocked from contributing creatively to the current situation, getting to a constructive decision, and learning from new information. If the attempt to control the emotional reaction breaks down, as it's prone to do, you're likely to end up behaving in a manner you later regret.

Make no mistake: the more the lower brain takes charge, the more you stress, and the more you stress, the more things go to hell in a handbasket. The seminal research on human performance by Wesley Sime at the University of Nebraska concluded that "the greater the stress, the greater the likelihood you'll make bad decisions." Communication will tank, aggression and escape behaviors will swamp your ability to work collaboratively, and the intolerance for ambiguity that stress produces will derail your capacity for creative problem solving. Sime found that in a climate of stress, survival goals tend to replace long-range considerations, making you much more likely to take risky alternatives.[9]

This is hardly the picture of peak performance. You can be sure that the lower brain has been set loose within a company when someone, in the heat of the moment, decides to vent their frustrations in an aggressive, finger-pointing email copied to everyone. This often has the effect of exciting the lower brains of other people in the department, either to collude with the person who initiated the email or to attack back. What follows is a cacophony of emotional negativity that undermines morale. You can thank the amygdala for this.

When a company makes an important hire, they're really hiring that person's higher brain and hoping it will function at full power, generating the level of intelligence that's needed to succeed. But when you put that brain into a high-pressure environment without teaching that person how to transcend stress, stress hormones are going to dampen brain power. Chronic stress means the stress response system is turned on nearly full time, releasing a steady stream of toxic hormones that dumb down the brain.

The fact is three out of four employees are stressed by at least one thing at work every week,[10] and a third of them are stressed to the extreme.[11] These numbers represent a drain on an organization's brainpower similar to a power brownout. It begs the question: how much more competitive and successful would an organization be if the power was restored?

Furthermore, depression and stress go hand in hand. Eighty percent of depressed cases are preceded by major stressful events[12] that cause a buildup of stress hormones.[13] This defeats the brain chemistry that keeps you on top of a situation. There are two PET scans from the Mayo Clinic that show the impact on brain function.* One scan shows a brain beleaguered by depression, and the other shows a healthy brain pulsing with activity. The scan of healthy brain activity looks like the massive array of light you see when flying over a metropolis on a dark night, while the depressed brain looks like the

---

* To view the Mayo Clinic scans, go to http://www.mayoclinic.com/health/medical/IM00356.

dim lights you might see when flying over farm country. The contrast is dramatic, revealing the significant decrease in brain activity that stress hormones cause. The lit-up scan represents the brain a VP is hoping she just hired when she offered someone a key position in her department. The dimly lit scan is what can happen over time to someone who hasn't learned how to transcend stress. Neurologically, a brain chronically under stress is simply incapable of sustaining peak performance day in, day out.

Stress Is Serious

As I said at the beginning of this chapter, stress is serious. It is life-threateningly serious and not something you should wait to address. Yet sadly, this is not what most people are doing. Surveys show that while nearly everyone agrees that stress makes us unhealthy and unproductive, 83 percent of us are doing nothing about it—an alarmingly high percentage.[14]

Why aren't people attending to stress? It's because people and companies have given up. They've accepted stress as the new normal. Try to sell a stress reduction program to a senior executive, and most likely he or she will groan and say good-bye. Such apathy stems from companies having spent millions of dollars in an effort to reduce stress, yet so far nothing has really worked. In fact, during the three decades conventional stress management has been around, stress levels have soared by 30 percent.[15]

If you have a problem with stress, it has a lot to do with the way genetics and a painful past have wired you for a hyperactive stress response system. The "painful past" part of it is the result of having had parents who also inherited the same stress-provoking gene, which can make for a stressful childhood. Increasingly, studies reveal that stress has more to do with genetic coding than with a person's job. Timothy Judge of the University of Notre Dame studied

594 twins, both identical and fraternal, some growing up together and others apart. He found that shared genes were four times more important in determining how they related to their job than was the job itself.[16] This suggests that work stress has a lot more to do with genes than researchers once thought. Two people can perform the exact same job under the same conditions, yet each person can have a completely different experience at work. One feels stressed, overwhelmed, and hates the job, while the other is happy and breezes through the day.

"This means," says Dr. Judge, "that stress may have less to do with the objective features of the environment than to the genetic 'code' of the individual."[17] This explains the failure of conventional stress management, which tends to relate to stress as outside pressures causing behavioral problems, when in fact stress-related behaviors are hardwired into the brain. Often, they happen in a knee-jerk fashion. Thus, any solution to the problem of stress requires rewiring the brain. And here is where neuroscience ran into its own brick wall. For a hundred years, science believed that the structure of the brain was fixed: in other words, the brain couldn't change. So if you were born with a hyperactive stress response system, making you a pessimist, you would probably die whining.

Well, science could not have been more wrong. As it turns out, the brain is highly malleable. Studies have shown that it's possible to change the brain so you can see, at least partially, if you are blind. The brain can physically remap its real estate to enable you to regain mobility that you lost to a stroke. And when it comes to a brain wired for stress, you can rewire those networks by changing your attitude. Literally! It's called neuroplasticity. It's the solution to stress that this book will help you achieve.

People have long recognized the effect that attitude can have on a person's ability to succeed. Thomas Jefferson said, "Nothing can stop the man with the right mental attitude . . . nothing on earth can help the man with the wrong mental attitude." We now know that there is a neurological basis for Jefferson's words. The right mental attitude is neuroplastic; it strengthens, expands, and activates neural networks that achieve goals. The stress hormones generated by the wrong mental attitude literally shrink these networks.

Over the years, when I have asked people in workshops and webinars if they think people can end stress, approximately 90 percent have said no. However, when I ask if they think humans can change their experience of life through a shift in attitude, nearly everyone answers yes. Most people don't understand the strong connection between attitude and stress, but there is a direct connection between attitude and the capacity of the brain to change in ways that quell stress reactions and expand brain capacity. It's a very simple algorithm: a change of attitude that changes your experience literally changes your brain structure.

Let's drill into that for a moment so we can see exactly what it means. Generating a new experience of life is a matter of attitude. And attitude shapes our experience. Change your attitude from judgmental to compassionate, from defensive to open, and you will experience people differently. Change your attitude from pessimistic to optimistic and you will experience problems differently; they turn into challenges you embrace instead of troubles you stress over. Your new attitude even helps you see the solution to the challenge. Change your attitude from worry and doubt to faith and trust and you will experience life in a completely new way. Change your attitude from fear to peace and you will end stress. Biologically, no fear means no stress reaction. If every day you practice shifting your attitude in this general direction, in just four to eight weeks your brain will rewire itself to quiet stress reactions and amplify higher-order brain function.[18]

If you still don't think attitude can wire the brain in ways that can kill you, and a shift in attitude can rewire the brain to save you, consider this: there is a direct connection between stress, attitude, and the health of chromosomes. Chromosomes hold the genes that rebuild and repair our bodies, and they are capped by organic structures called telomeres. Telomeres are responsible for keeping our chromosomes healthy and working properly. They act much in the same way that tape binds together the ends of a frayed rope. If these caps deteriorate, our chromosomes begin to rearrange themselves and produce abnormal cells that can cause cancer. Additionally, frayed or shortened telomeres make healthy cells age faster, causing a host of aging-related diseases that shorten life span.

What causes telomeres to fray and shorten? The answer is stress hormones. Stress hormones shorten telomeres. The length of telomeres is directly related to the amount of stress you have been under and the number of years you've endured stress.[19] Neuropsychologist Elissa Epel and Nobel Prize laureate Elizabeth Blackburn, both of the University of California at San Francisco, studied mothers caring for severely disabled children.[20] The daily demands on these women are stressful to the point of overwhelming, and the study found that a high percentage of the women had shortened telomeres. The research found that there was in excess of ten years of extra aging in their blood cells, which Blackburn said was actually a conservative estimate. But not all of these mothers exhibited shortened telomeres. The telomeres of mothers who had cultivated a positive, peaceful attitude were still intact and supporting healthy chromosomes. As a result, they were likely to live a much longer and healthier life. "I have a great attitude," one of the mothers said, "because that's what I give myself to do. That's my goal, to have a good attitude. Because if I didn't have a good attitude, who'd want to talk to me?"[21] She accepted what she couldn't change and met the challenge of changing herself. The attitude she cultivated transcended her circumstances, and as a result, her telomeres were still intact.

Dr. Steven Cole of the University of California at Los Angeles states that "both our experience of meaning and purpose in life seem to be recurrent themes that associate tightly with favorable molecular changes."[22] Increasingly, the evidence reveals that human biology, from your brain structure right down to your chromosomes, is shaped by your mental state.

Even more amazing is that it takes relatively little time for a change in attitude to effect a positive change in your biology. "Changing the way you think about and relate to the world for two to three months," states Cole, "is sufficient to actually generate a noticeable effect at the molecular level."[23] The world for these mothers can be defined as all the circumstances they would never completely control, whereas attitude was the one and only thing over which they had total control. For the mothers who cultivated a positive and peaceful attitude, it made all the difference—biologically, psychologically, and spiritually.

In addition, the research of Edward Nelson of the University of California at Irvine suggests that damaged telomeres can be repaired. In a study of cervical cancer survivors, Dr. Nelson found that when these women participated in psychological counseling that reduced the stress response, the length of their telomeres increased.[24]

We all want to live longer, healthier, happier lives. These findings have established that it all begins with the quality of your attitude. The maxim that "attitude is everything" is not just a slogan on a motivational poster—it's a medical prescription for a better life.

From Fear to Peace

The change in attitude that generates the powerful effects of neuroplasticity is the fundamental shift from fear to peace. It is called *positive neuroplasticity*, and it is the key to the Good Life, which is a life of being well and doing well on your way to flourishing. This book presents fear and peace not in spiritual terms, but from a neurological perspective.

Neurologically, fear is the trigger that sets off stress reactions. It's the fear of danger. For modern human beings, rarely is the stress response system triggered by a real and present danger, such as a rattlesnake. More often, stress reactions are triggered by psychological fear that mistakes a coiled rope for a snake. "We human beings are smart enough to generate all sorts of stressful events purely in our heads . . . all linked to mere thoughts," writes Robert Sapolsky of Stanford University School of Medicine.[25] These thoughts excite upsetting emotions that produce a perception of threat, sending the brain and mind into an uproar. In short, you paint yourself into a stressful corner with your thoughts, but awareness of the mental pattern that trapped you is what gets you out of that tight corner. Awareness creates a kind of pattern interrupt within the brain that puts things on pause for a moment and presents you with the opportunity to choose a more positive course of action—one that preserves your peace of mind. When you bring a stressful thought pattern safely into awareness, where its illusion can be challenged and dispelled, a new memory is formed that inhibits the old conditioned response.[26] Conscious awareness excites a neuroplastic process that strengthens a specific neural pathway made of gamma-aminobutyric acid (GABA) fibers. This neural pathway projects down to the amygdala, the brain's fear center, and secretes peptides that extinguish fear reactions: no fear, no stress reaction. And as we've seen, no stress reaction, no loss of brain power. The higher brain comes online and can now assist you in making an intelligent choice. It turns out that, neurologically, inner peace is the most intelligent choice, because inner peace facilitates the brain chemistry and structure that promote intelligence.

Peace begins where stress ends. So let's define peace in neurological terms. In terms of your brain, peace represents neural networks wiring and firing together to sustain the proverbial calm under siege that enables you to relate to a problem fearlessly, analyze it intelligently, engage it creatively, and make the best available choice or decision in a given situation. Essentially, being stress free is a dynamically peaceful mind-set. Practice shifting your experience from fear to peace, and in a few weeks, positive neuroplastic change will occur.

This shift from fear to peace is made by accentuating simple principles. It's letting go of fear. It's refusing to believe worried, pessimistic, and stress-provoking thoughts. It's being present, here and now, living each moment fully. It's trusting the process of life as it unfolds, changing what you can, and accepting what you can't change. It's being open, honest, and flexible. It's grounding yourself in the authentic person you are instead of chasing some ideal of who you, or others, think you should be. It's having faith in yourself. It's pursuing what you love with a sense of purpose, perpetually anticipating positive outcomes. It's having unconditional positive regard and empathy for the people in your life. It's listening to them better, judging them less, forgiving them more, and being kinder.

In referring to these principles as "simple," I don't mean to imply that they are easy to attain. But they don't need to be hard, either. Like a garden, principles require cultivation. Cultivate even a few of these qualities, and they will eventually come together to form a dynamically peaceful attitude. Empower a dynamically peaceful attitude in your daily life, and within a matter of weeks that new attitude will become neuroplastic, producing the brain structure that generates more success in your endeavors, more joy in your work, more love in your relationships, more peace in your day, and more spring in your step.

My think tank and I took all these findings and built a model to teach people how to end stress based on cognitive, emotional, and attitudinal processes that facilitate neuroplasticity. The training model teaches a set of tools and processes that gradually build into a practice that integrates into your daily life. The training is delivered over eight weeks, reflecting the outside range of how long neuroplasticity takes. This book has reconfigured the training model into a program that you can easily follow. If you practice the tools and processes with consistency, your brain will begin to change to end stress. How long it takes depends on the degree to which you practice. If you don't practice, the information in this book will still take you part way up the mountain, but forming a daily practice from the tools and processes can take you to the summit.

Practice is taking the right step repeatedly until that step takes you effortlessly, almost automatically, in the direction you want to go. You now understand the neurological importance of peace and its power to generate the brain function to deliver an optimal life experience—in your career, in your personal life, in yourself. After all is said and done, peace is what matters in life.

Practice takes discipline, and discipline is simply remembering what you want and choosing it. The discipline of peace gets easier the more you choose it, simply because peace makes everything easier. Making the shift from stress to peace is the energetic shift from feeling poorly to feeling alive and healthy. It is the mental shift from feeling worried, lackluster, and disconnected to being clear, bright, and resonant.

So, let's get started. If you haven't yet read the section called How to Use This Book in the introduction, please do so now. Otherwise, turn to chapter 2 to begin Step 1, which facilitates neuroplastic change by bringing your pattern of stress into greater awareness.

BUILDING AWARENESS

The Insight That Ends Stress as You Know It

2

The Stress Assessment: Exposing Your Blind Side

The first step in becoming stress free is building *awareness* about your pattern of stress, beginning with a self-assessment of your current level of stress. Uncovering the areas of your life where stress raises its ugly head is the first step in making a change. Stress-provoking behaviors habituate to the point that you may not even see them, much less regard them as stress. As Alan Watts once said, "Normally we do not so much look at things as overlook them," and what we don't see can blindside us.[1]

A cardiologist once told me that it's not uncommon for patients recovering from a recent heart event to say, "I didn't know I was that stressed," even though most of these people were routinely working fifty to sixty hours a week in high-pressure jobs and hadn't taken a real vacation in years. You can become so adapted to a stressful life that it seems normal. Some people even wear stress as a badge of honor. They see themselves as warriors who are effectively managing the daily demands and pressures at home and work, until suddenly, one day, their face droops from an acute ischemic stroke, or their chest tightens with a pain that makes it hard to breathe. My friend the cardiologist says if these people are really lucky, the symptoms resolve on their own, providing a wake-up call that the afflicted answer by slowing down. If they're really unlucky, they die or face paralysis.

This book is designed to help make you one of the lucky ones. It all begins with becoming conscious of the signs and symptoms of stress so you don't get blindsided.

The following is your stress assessment. I recommend that you take it right now, checking off any statements that describe your experience of life recently. Keep your answers current (within the last week or month), take your time, and be totally honest with yourself. Facts are friendly when brought out of the dark into the light, even when we don't like what the light reveals. Left in the dark, unpleasant facts tend to torment and undermine us. But in the light of day, they become a kind of grace that reveals to us what we need to learn and change in order to live, love, and succeed fully.

Each of the statements you checked reflects a sign or symptom of stress. It doesn't matter how many you checked. This isn't a test that gives you a score that equates to a diagnosis. It's a self-assessment that gives you a feeling or sense of where stress impacts your life. It also increases your awareness of the different ways in which stress manifests, since you may not have previously equated some of the items with stress. What matters as you review the results is your willingness to look clearly at the signs and symptoms you checked and become aware of the ways in which each one thwarts you.

After taking the assessment, read back to yourself the items you checked. Do this in a conversational manner, as if you were describing your stress level to a trusted friend. Reviewing your results in this way should give you a good idea, intuitively, of the trouble stress is causing in your life. When you're finished reviewing your assessment, check the description below that you think relates to your level of stress:

STRESS ASSESSMENT TOOL

O I get less and less pleasure from activities that I used to enjoy.	O I experience fatigue most days and at times become exhausted.
O I have trouble making decisions.	O I'm having difficulty getting to sleep because I can't quiet down, or I'm sleeping more than usual and don't want to get out of bed.
O My memory and concentration are not as good as they used to be.	O I feel less confident about my ability to handle my personal problems.
O Simple things feel burdensome or difficult to accomplish.	O At times I feel overwhelmed and unable to control the important things in my life.
O I have a shorter fuse these days. I'm more impatient, more on edge, and more easily frustrated or annoyed.	O I lose track of little things, such as where I put my keys.
O I experience upsetting emotions such as fear, paranoia, dejection, worry, or pessimism to a greater degree or for prolonged periods.	O I worry over things I can't control.
O I criticize my significant other more, tend to ruminate on the flaws in our relationship, bicker more, and blame my partner for our problems.	O At times, my agitation or frustration can reach the point that I bang on my desk with my fist, throw things, shout, or act out in some other way.
O I've become less social. I find myself wishing that people, including friends and family, would stop bothering me.	O My interest in sex has decreased.
O I eat more to cope with my emotional state, or I have lost my appetite.	O I get sick more often than I think I should, catching colds and flu. I have developed or worry about developing serious health risks.
O My use of alcohol, tobacco, or other substances has increased in part to relieve stress.	O I have tension headaches, gastro-intestinal problems, muscle tension in the back, neck, or jaw, or all of the above.

➤ **This worksheet is available for download at theendofstressbook.com/worksheets.**

☐ Extreme stress
☐ High stress
☐ Medium stress
☐ Low stress
☐ Stress free

The Neurological Trouble
Behind These Questions

The statements below (in **bold**) are from a case study of a typical stress assessment for a person experiencing extreme stress. The statements this person checked are followed by a neurobiological explanation of how that particular problem affects the brain.

I get less and less pleasure from activities that I used to enjoy. Neurobiological explanation: A stress hormone called adrenal glucocorticoid interacts with serotonin receptors in the brain when stress is high or chronic. This interferes with our capacity to experience pleasure and remain motivated.[2] Serotonin levels that are consistently out of balance produce the brain chemistry that leads to depression.

I have trouble making decisions. Neurobiological explanation: An episode of uncontrollable stress impairs decision-making in rats for several days, rendering them unable to reliably identify the larger of two rewards.[3] Additionally, the greater the stress, the greater the likelihood we'll make bad decisions.[4]

My memory and concentration are not as good as they used to be. Neurobiological explanation: Acute psychological stress reduces working and prospective memory and reallocates neural resources away from executive function networks.[5] That's a technical way of saying stress causes memory lapse, attention deficit, and an inability of higher-brain networks to carry out a plan.

Simple things feel burdensome or difficult to accomplish. Neurobiological explanation: Stress hormones can elevate dopamine levels in the brain, creating a decline in cognitive performance.[6] When cognitive performance declines, even easy tasks can become difficult to manage. Also, stress can cause us to stop looking for new ways to approach old tasks, even when an old way fails. Behavior tends to habituate when the brain is under stress and the brain locks into doing the same unproductive thing over and over. This eventually results in our abandoning the task altogether.[7]

I have a shorter fuse these days. I'm more impatient, more on edge, and more easily frustrated or annoyed. And I experience upsetting emotions such as fear, paranoia, dejection, worry, or pessimism to a greater degree or for prolonged periods. Neurobiological explanation: Stress is closely associated with fear. When we are afraid that we are at risk, the brain shifts to survival mode. The amygdala, the brain's fear center, activates fight, flight, or freeze, which switches the brain's emotional set point to negative. We become aggressive, angry, or defensive. This is because evolution determined that a hostile stance was a better survival strategy in the event of a threat than peace and loving kindness. This is quite true, of course, if we're faced with a grizzly bear. But few of us are ever threatened by a wild animal. Our plunge into an edgy emotional state is the result of stressing over an imagined threat that often doesn't exist.

I criticize my significant other more, tend to ruminate on the flaws in our relationship, bicker more frequently, and blame

my partner for our problems. Neurobiological explanation: Fifteen years of research by Benjamin Karney of the University of California at Los Angeles found that the greater the stress, the more reactive we'll be to the normal ups and downs at home.[8] The more stressed we are, the more we and our partner will argue, criticize, blame, and withhold affection from each other. We're much more likely to judge the relationship as negative and blame our loved one for a problem, not realizing the way stress is distorting how we see the relationship. In addition, stress hormones add to the growing alienation by lowering sex drive.

I've become less social. I find myself wishing that people, including friends and family, would stop bothering me. Neurobiological explanation: People tend to isolate when they are chronically stressed. In fact, social isolation plays a major role in people's inability to deal with stress.[9] Type-A personalities experience extreme stress and tend to generate little or no social support to help buffer them at the end of a stressful day. They actually shun support.[10]

I eat more to cope with my emotional state, or I have lost my appetite. Neurobiological explanation: Stress makes about two-thirds of people hyperphagic (eat more) and the rest hypophagic (eat less). Glucocorticoid is the stress hormone that stimulates appetite, and it can take hours for glucocorticoids to be cleared from the bloodstream.[11] During that time, it's not uncommon to put away a bag of potato chips, a soft drink, and a chocolate cookie.

My use of alcohol, tobacco, or other substances has increased, in part to relieve stress. Neurobiological explanation: Stress hormones trigger substance abuse[12] and cause a greater chance of relapse in recovering alcoholics.[13]

I experience fatigue most days and at times become exhausted. Neurobiological explanation: During a stressful day, the brain's stress response system is turned on almost nonstop. Stress hormones are dumped into the blood system, which in turn accelerates heart rate and respiration and activates the sympathetic nervous system. The sympathetic nervous system mobilizes fight, flight, or freeze. The system expends a lot of energy and we become fatigued. By the end of the day, we wind up exhausted.[14]

I'm having difficulty getting to sleep because I can't quiet down, or I'm sleeping more than usual and don't want to get out of bed. Neurobiological explanation: Studies show that poor sleepers tend to have higher levels of stress hormones in their bloodstream. If the day has been particularly stressful, the likelihood is we'll have little sleep at night. Stress hormones not only decrease the total amount of sleep we get but can compromise the quality of whatever sleep we end up getting.[15] The result is that we return to work the next day with even less energy than the day before.

I feel less confident about my ability to handle my personal problems. Neurobiological explanation: For people who feel that the majority or all of the above statements apply to them, it is not surprising that they would also feel incapable of handling their personal problems. How could anyone feel confident in their ability to handle problems when their brain is malfunctioning to this degree? The buildup of stress hormones makes us depressed, which lowers self-esteem, and we lose the brain chemistry that enables us to stay on top of a situation.[16]

It All Can Change

All of these problems are reversible. In the chapters that follow, you will learn how to build the attitude that transcends stress, secures your health and well-being, and lights up your higher brain to function fully. The stress assessment you just took is not static. It's a tool you can use over time to gauge your progress in alleviating the neurological problems I've just cited. Tracking your improvement is enormously motivating. You can download a copy of the Stress Assessment Tool at theendofstressbook.com.

Following is an example of someone who is learning to transcend extreme stress. The items listed represent issues she might have checked during the initial stress assessment. Alleviating these issues is a result of practicing the tools and processes described in this book. You can see through the example how your life can improve, week by week, as a result of practicing the tools.

After Two Weeks: The Following Four Items Initially Checked Are No Longer Checked

- ☑ I worry over things I can't control.
- ☑ I have a shorter fuse these days. I'm more impatient, more on edge, and more easily frustrated or annoyed.
- ☑ I experience upsetting emotions such as fear, paranoia, dejection, worry, or pessimism to a greater degree or for prolonged periods.
- ☑ At times, my agitation or frustration can reach the point that I bang on my desk with my fist, throw things, shout, or act out in some other way.

With these four items no longer checked, she would now be more aware of stress-provoking thoughts and actively working at not believing these thoughts. As a result, she would be less worried and less prone to the old upsets. This positive change in mood builds into a greater sense of self-control. She's beginning to feel more at peace.

After Four Weeks:
The Following Five More Items Initially Checked Are No Longer Checked

☑ I get less and less pleasure from activities that I used to enjoy.
☑ I have trouble making decisions.
☑ My memory and concentration are not as good as they used to be.
☑ I experience fatigue most days and at times become exhausted.
☑ I'm having difficulty getting to sleep because I can't quiet down, or I'm sleeping more than usual and don't want to get out of bed.

Now four weeks into a consistent practice, the person in this example is enjoying work more and feeling clearheaded throughout the day instead of distracted and fatigued. Memory and concentration have improved, and she is accomplishing more. Her energy level is higher, and she is feeling her vitality return. The decline in stress hormones in her system means she is sleeping easier and waking up feeling refreshed instead of beleaguered.

Eight weeks has come and gone since she first took the stress assessment, and she has been consistent in practicing the tools and processes. Now, only one of the initially selected items is checked. As a result, this person is functioning at or near the top of her game at work. Her relationships, both at home and with friends, have become more enjoyable and fulfilling. Constructive habits are replacing destructive habits. In short, this person's life has been transformed through a fundamental shift in attitude that rewired her brain for the Good Life.

She has become basically stress free. The key to this shift was positive neuroplasticity. This example is representative of the extraordinary shift that ordinary people are capable of making.

Belief Creates the Actual Fact

The father of American psychology, William James, said, "If you can change your mind, you can change your life." He said, "Belief creates the actual fact." One way to reinforce a belief is to visualize that belief coming true. So imagine a breakthrough with stress and anxiety for yourself. Take a moment and believe that you, too, can make the changes to strike unfavorable items from your stress assessment list. Let your imagination make the possibility of change real for a moment.

- Reflect for a moment on how you want to feel as you work. Now imagine feeling this way.
- Reflect on the state of mind you want to sustain throughout the day. Imagine yourself achieving this state of mind.
- Reflect on how you want to be with your coworkers. Imagine relating to people in this way.
- How do you want your brain to perform as you work? Imagine performing at the top of your game.
- How do you want to feel physically each and every day? Imagine feeling this way.
- Reflect on how you want to be with your loved ones at the end of the day. Imagine being this way at home.

Now pull together everything you've just imagined and believe it is in the process of coming true. "Belief creates the actual fact," so believe it. Believe this change is coming.

A Tool for Starting Your Day

Let's start using the first tool. It's called "Starting the Day in Quiet." This tool is an antidote to the frenetic, early morning rush out of the door. It encourages you to set aside five minutes first thing each morning to consciously frame a dynamically positive and peaceful mind-set for meeting the day's challenges with confidence. A quiet and conscious mind-set is not how people typically start their day. Most of us jump out of bed, gulp down a cup of coffee or two, feed and dress the kids, get ready ourselves, and then drive straight into the morning traffic jam. This kind of routine is bound to frame the day in stress. The Starting the Day in Quiet Tool avoids the downward spiral into stress by helping you consciously evoke a higher frame of mind to shape the new day. At the end of this chapter, you will find the step-by-step process for using this tool.

The idea at the center of this tool has been with us since antiquity. It's captured in the Latin phrase *carpe diem*, which, in modern times, has come to mean "seize the day." The phrase comes from a poem by Horace, Rome's leading lyric poet during the time of Augustus. In Latin, *carpe* literally means "to pluck the fruit," and *diem* means "the day." Thus, for Romans the phrase meant "Pluck the day, for it is ripe," and these words became a creed. The modern translation—seize the day—can become your creed that frames each day consciously by asserting the power of attitude. It might strike you as implausible that significant change could come from setting aside five minutes each morning to sit quietly and set your attitude, but when participants in my seminars make this practice part of their morning routine, they report that the rest of the day goes much more smoothly.

There is a neurological reason to start each new day by asserting the power of attitude. It's because evolution set the brain's default to survival mode, which was necessary when we human beings lived in the wilderness and survival was an issue every day. Of course, we no longer live in the wild, but evolution hasn't had the millennia it takes to do a brain makeover. Thus, on waking each day, you can count on your brain's survival system to be on its toes, ready, willing, and able to flood you with stress hormones at the first sign of trouble, which

9.9 times out of 10 is the lower brain's misperception of trouble. You have to consciously reset the default or you'll be prone to stress reactions that day.

Your Practice This Week

Start the day in quiet in a conscious manner, using the simple process delineated in the exercise below.

Tools

Starting the Day in Quiet

Read this page each day until you are clear on how to apply this process.

- Wake up fifteen or so minutes ahead of the rush.
- Sit quietly in a place where you won't be disturbed. At first, you can do this exercise while you're waiting for the coffee to brew, as long as you won't be disturbed. Later, as you get into the flow of it, you might move to someplace more conducive to peace.
- Close your eyes or gaze downward. Tilt your head toward your heart and follow your breathing. Feel each breath as it softens your heart and opens it wider.
- Feel each breath enlivening your brain with oxygen, waking you up.
- Now feel appreciation for the gift of another day of life.
- Feel gratitude for another day with the people you love.
- Set your intention to have a rewarding and productive day.
- Commit yourself today to being positive and at peace on the inside, regardless of what happens on the outside. Feel the power of your attitude seizing hold of the day and shaping it into a great one.
- Recall what William James said: "If you can change your mind, you can change your life," and "Belief creates the actual fact."

Materials You Can Download

You can use your smartphone to download the free app to scan the QR tags for downloading audio files to your smartphone. Or you can go to theendofstressbook.com to download the book's worksheets, tools, and audio files.

3

The Awareness That Extinguishes Stress

So far, I've established that peace is neurological power: a dynamically peaceful mind-set, as neuroscience defines it, is key in generating a powerful brain. I've also established that stress is psychological fear. It's happening *in* you far more than *to* you. But the validity of something always sinks in more deeply when demonstrated empirically through your own experience.

Let's start with my statement that peace is power and see where the dynamic of peace makes you powerful in your life. To do this, take out a piece of paper and, without looking at the table that follows, list ten to twelve qualities that identify your experience when you're at the top of your game: in the flow, in the zone, making things happen, sailing along toward achieving something meaningful. Take your time and reflect on how this powerful experience felt.

Now look at the table. This list is typical of how people define the experience of being at the top of their game when I've performed this exercise in seminars over the years. Look it over and compare it to your list. Add any entries from this list to your list if they also apply to your experience.

Creative	Decisive
Energized	Stimulated
Engaged	Calm
Confident	At peace
Quick	Connected
Productive	See the big picture
Celebratory	Connecting the dots
Communicative	Passionate
Positive	Collaborative
At choice	Impactful
Fearless	Reflecting
Listen better	Creative

This list of qualities that describe you at the top of your game can also be said to represent a specific kind of attitude. My human performance firm has been doing this exercise for nine years, and the quality people most often cite is feeling calm and clear-minded, or at peace. Peace is the very foundation of all the qualities people list. Together, these attributes form a dynamically positive and peaceful attitude, which is the polar opposite of the fight, flight, and freeze reaction that stress produces. Some people think that peace represents complacency or passivity or losing one's edge. Few, if any of us, think of peace as the gateway to cerebral power. Yet this list hardly fits the description of complacency. The fact that people can come up with a list that equates a dynamically peaceful attitude with peak performance means they understand it, perhaps more than they realize. It's not necessarily something you need to learn; it's something you need to accentuate in your daily life until it becomes your everyday experience.

You can start right now. I have compiled a list of attributes that pinpoint a dynamically peaceful attitude, drawn from a composite of the qualities people most often cite as the ones they experience when performing at the top of their game. I converted the list into a tool for transcending stress called Attributes of a Dynamically Peaceful Attitude. I invite you to select three qualities that you would like to accentuate throughout this week, starting today. Look at each quality you select, one at a time, and remember how it feels to be this way. Then make that past experience real, as if it were happening now. You might surprise yourself with how vividly you can recall this experience, but even a glimpse of it is enough. Invoking each quality in this way sets the change in motion as you go about your day. You can trust that you will naturally find ways to accentuate all three qualities. Maintaining awareness of what you want to accentuate will lead the way to a change in your experience.

Dynamically Peaceful Audio:
A three-and-a-half-minute audio in which Don describes the Dynamically Peaceful Attitude.

http://www.beyondword.com/theendofstress/tag1_Dynamically
-Peaceful.mp3

These attributes describe your state of mind, not external conditions. They hold the potential to make you larger than external conditions. That's enormous personal power. Sadly, this isn't the everyday experience of most people. As I cited in the introduction, every week, three out of four people are stressed by at least one thing at work,[1] and a third of them are stressed to the extreme nearly every day.[2] A brain under stress is incapable of sustaining you at the top of your game; stress makes a brain rapidly devolve into the opposite experience. So let's look at the second premise that says stress is psychological fear, meaning it's happening in you far more than to you. Let's see if this is true in your experience.

Flip over the sheet of paper you just used to create your list in relation to you at the top of your game. Take a few moments and, without looking at the following stress list, make a list of ten or

ATTRIBUTES OF A DYNAMICALLY PEACEFUL ATTITUDE[3]

Check three qualities listed below that you want to strengthen.

O Calm	O Resilient
O A clear sense of personal power and the integrity to assert your power without overpowering others	O Faith in the face of adversity
O Unafraid	O Trust in the process
O Unhurried	O Joy in the challenge
O Free of worry	O Empathic
O Self-confident	O A willingness to forgive
O Creative	O A disinterest in judging or condemning
O Open-minded, receptive, and accepting	O A felt connection with one's own heart, with others, and with life itself
O A curiosity that is fully present	O An enduring sense of the whole that transcends the fragments
O Energetic	O A sense of the sacred

This worksheet is available for download at theendofstressbook.com/worksheets.

twelve words or phrases that come to mind when you reflect on the condition of stress as it applies to your life.

Once you've done this, look at the following list, which reflects what people cited most often in workshops and keynotes I've conducted. Take a moment and compare your list to this one. Feel free to add any entries from this list to your list that also apply to your experience.

Stress as We Know It

Depressed	Confusion
Traffic jams	Anger
Feeling stuck	Defensive
My boss	Memory lapses
My team	Emotionally negative
Discouraged	Trouble concentrating
Feeling defeated	Withdrawn
Long meetings	Loss of control
Family demands	Overwhelm
Fear of failing	Losing sleep
To-do list	Overeating
Anxiety	Abusing alcohol

Consider this list as a whole. It does not represent the life anyone would choose to live, yet it's staggering to consider that it is the life many people are living. In seminars, I ask people to go over their stress list and ascertain which of the entries are internal in nature, reflecting their state of mind, and which entries are external factors that circumstances impose. I invite you to do the same exercise with your list. Go over each item and decide whether it represents an internal state of mind or an imposing external condition.

Next is the stress list I just presented, with each item marked according to how the participants evaluated the item, internal versus external. The items marked with (I) were assessed by the group to be internal. Those that are marked with (E) were initially assessed as external, while those marked with (B) were assessed as both external and internal. You can see from this list that the overwhelming number of items were evaluated as internal reactions.

Stress: Internal or External?

Depressed (I)	Confusion (I)
Traffic jams (B)	Anger (I)
Feeling stuck (I)	Defensive (I)
My boss (E)	Memory lapses (I)
My team (E)	Emotionally negative (I)
Discouraged (I)	Trouble concentrating (I)
Feeling defeated (I)	Withdrawn (I)
Long meetings (E)	Loss of control (I)
Family demands (B)	Overwhelm (I)
Fear of failing (I)	Losing sleep (I)
To-do list (B)	Overeating (I)
Anxiety (I)	Abusing alcohol (I)

When I've asked people to take a closer look at items they classified as external, they often decide that most can be defined as both external and internal (marked with a B). For example, a traffic jam is both the backup of cars and the way you relate to the backup. The same can be said of an unmanageable to-do list. Try using the Serenity Prayer to shift how stressed you sometimes feel about your to-do list. The prayer states, "Grant me the serenity to accept the things I cannot change; courage to change the things I can; and wisdom to know the difference." I invite you to look at your to-do list and, after reciting this prayer, consider letting go of items you know you can't possibly address, at least not any time soon. Then prioritize the items you can address, and see what happens to your stress level.

By looking at your own stress list, you can begin to see how much of what excites a debilitating stress reaction is happening in you far more than to you. When we stop and take a breath, we begin to see the choice that now confronts us, which is to either continue to be caught in a debilitating stress reaction or take responsibility for our mental state. This is the first step in changing our brain to transform our experience, and there's no getting around this step.

This is not to say that losing your job, being diagnosed with a serious illness, or having your home go into foreclosure isn't happening to you. Of course it is. Yet, even in the most dire of circumstances, we can still effect transformational change. Viktor Frankl is an example of the extraordinary capacity of an ordinary man to transcend even a hopeless situation. Frankl was an Austrian neurologist and psychiatrist and a Holocaust survivor. He spent three years in Auschwitz and Dachau, where he was used as slave labor. His wife and all of but one member of his immediate family died at the hands of the Nazis. In the camps, Frankl took it upon himself to organize general medical care for the prisoners as best he could. He also set up a suicide watch unit. In treating the men, he found one consistent factor that predicted who was more likely to survive the horrendous physical and psychological abuse in the camps: attitude. He wrote, "What was really needed was a fundamental change in our attitude toward life. We had to learn ourselves and, furthermore, we had to teach the despairing men that it did not really matter what we expected from life, but rather what life expected from us."[4]

Frankl went on to establish a school of psychology called Logotherapy and to write a book on his experiences in the concentration camps entitled *Man's Search for Meaning*, which the Library of Congress determined to be one of the ten most influential books in America.[5] Frankl was often invited to give lectures as a visiting professor at major universities around the world, including Harvard. It was common during the Q&A at the end of his lecture for someone in the audience to praise him as a great and enlightened man who was able to transcend the horror he faced in ways most people could not. Frankl adamantly refuted these accolades as self-demeaning and an abdication of the personal responsibility to choose one's own way, regardless of circumstances. He asserted that the attitude that sustained him during his ordeal was potential in all of us. "We must never forget," Frankl wrote, "that we may also find meaning in life even when . . . facing a fate that cannot be changed. For what then matters is to bear witness to the uniquely human potential at its best, which is to transform a personal tragedy into a triumph."[6]

During the last economic downturn, we all heard of people confronted with losing their jobs and their homes in foreclosure. Some faced pre-existing health problems without a company medical plan to pay for treatment. I understood much of what these people were going through, as I had been through it myself. Actually, I had faced all three calamities at the same time. Twenty-five years ago my life was engulfed by what I call my perfect storm of stress. I had a high-powered job at Stanford Medical School, working with world-class people, and I was at the height of my career to that point. But within the course of one week my entire life was turned upside down. At the beginning of the week I was fired from that job, and by the end of the week I was diagnosed with a brain tumor. I was married with four small children and had a variable-rate mortgage payment that had gone through the roof, which unemployment compensation or disability insurance couldn't possibly cover. To make matters worse, my marriage was on the rocks. For years I'd been wedded to my career more than to my wife, and the stress of this situation only widened the cracks in our marriage.

How would you react to this storm of stress? Would you raise an angry fist to heaven and shout WHY ME? I did that for a time. Would you roll up into a ball of fear and hide from reality? I did that as well. Or would you look this situation square in the eye and say, "Wow, what an opportunity to realize my 'uniquely human potential . . . to transform a personal tragedy into a triumph,'" as Viktor Frankl did? I most definitely did not start out like that.

The only fortunate thing about my situation was that the brain tumor was slow growing, allowing me to wait six weeks to get on the busy schedule of the best neurosurgeon in the area. But this also meant I had a lot of time to ruminate over my calamity. The surgeon had told me to prepare myself psychologically for having a paralyzed face, being half deaf, needing a walker to navigate across the room, along with a warning about other frightening complications that brain surgery could create. It terrified me. I couldn't imagine anyone would hire me in that physical condition, which meant my career was over, my family was headed for the poorhouse, and I would die a failure. Every night for the first few weeks I would wake up in the wee hours of the morning and stare out a window into the dark, overwhelmed by fear. Then one night I reached a point where I questioned which was worse: the enormous set of problems happening to me or the one enormous problem of fear happening in me. Somehow I managed to raise my mind above the fear and stress to a place of peace and quiet. In the calm atmosphere that ensued, I recognized that things would be materially better for me if I could shift the way my mind was constantly painting me into a corner of gloom and doom and foster an attitude of faith. I didn't have a clue how things could turn to the good, but I could see how, at the very least, this shift in attitude would make me feel so much better. I decided, then and there, to work at letting go of fear and stress and to strengthen my willingness to be at peace and have faith as I faced whatever I had to face that day.

Part of my termination package required me to stay on for a month to help the department transition. It was an unusual arrangement, and I hated having to go back to work each day, but my new attitude actually changed how I felt about it. Now I just wanted to do a good job and leave things in good order. When I returned to work, I noticed that the usual stressors didn't bother me. I was much better able to take things in stride. I had a clearer sense of what I could accomplish and what I couldn't, what I controlled and what I didn't, and I focused on areas where I could make a difference. I was even friendly to people I'd previously perceived as adversaries and blamed for my demise.

I stopped believing fearful, judgmental thoughts and perceptions, primarily because I wanted to give my mind every chance to heal in the hope it might heal my brain. I worked right up to a few days before the surgery, and during that entire time, as I recall, I did not entertain one negative thought. I discovered that choosing to be at peace wasn't as hard as I thought. Actually, it made everything easier.

My change in attitude changed the outcome. The surgery was a complete success, sparing me a life of disability. Medical science would now describe the positive outcome as the result of my positive mental state achieving the mind-body connection that can change a medical prognosis. I actually was "un-fired." The dean opened the way for me to apply for a position in another department. The chairman who eventually hired me told me he wanted my positive attitude on his team. Eventually, I left Stanford and pursued a whole new direction, one more aligned with my heart. None of this would have happened had I remained stressed and frightened.

There was nothing heroic about me. It was simply a decision I made to stop suffering by my own hand. I worked with a number of people during the economic downturn who came to the same conclusion, and, as a result, regained the emotional strength and creative thinking that enabled them to land on their feet.

We have more control over stress and fear than we might imagine. We have the power to direct ourselves to be at peace, regardless of circumstances. Peace arises naturally out of the decision not to be afraid, which is a decision to use our higher brain instead of allowing our lower brain to use us. Most items on the stress list are some form of psychological fear. They're generated by the lower brain function that can't tell the difference between a real and present danger and one you imagined. The lower brain sets off a stress reaction if either one is present. In short, psychological fear is the mind making up emergencies that the brain believes are real. The great French essayist Michel de Montaigne captured it when he said, "My life has been full of terrible misfortunes, most of which never happened."[7]

There was a study at Cornell that determined how many of our imagined calamities actually do happen.[8] In this study, subjects were asked to write down their worries over a two-week period and then identify which ones actually occurred. The study found that 85 percent of what subjects worried about never happened. With the 15 percent that did happen, 79 percent of subjects handled the matter better than they expected. These findings suggest that we have nothing to worry about almost 97 percent of the time. The prescription is to stop believing our worried, fearful thoughts. If we could get a handle on the fearful thinking that is habitually, often unconsciously, and sometimes incessantly going on in our heads, we could end stress as we know it. This book offers a simple set of tools that can start you on the road to busting psychological fear.

In seminars, I employ a guided process to help people drill down into a recent stress event, tapping their imagination to make the stressful experience as vivid as possible. Next, I have them notice first their *mental reaction*, then their *emotional reaction*, and then their *physical reaction*. Finally, I ask them to take note of any *change in attitude* that may have occurred as they disengaged from the stressful event. Using a scale of 0 to 100, where 100 indicates an extreme reaction and 0 indicates no reaction, participants assess how intense their reactions were in each of the four categories (mental, emotional, physical, and change in attitude). Invariably, people assign a very high number to their mental reaction during a stressful event, ranging from 85 to 100. Not far behind is a strong emotional reaction, but stressful thinking usually wins the top rating. Physical reactions generally lag behind emotions. Additionally, nearly everyone reports a decline in their attitude as a result of the event.

Here's the point the data makes: turning off the stress response system has more to do with changing your own negative, stress-provoking thinking than with changing your circumstances. Clearly, stress is an internal matter, and so is peace. Both begin with your own thoughts and then extend outward. It is from an anxious, worried mind that a stressful perception of the world arises. Equally, it is from a dynamically positive and peaceful state of mind that a stress-free experience is attained.

The Thought Awareness Tool

There's a tool that can facilitate a shift from stress to peace and reverse the damage an unhealthy mind-set can cause. It's called the Thought Awareness Tool: *I could see peace instead of this.*[9]

The first step in utilizing this tool is to be aware of stressful, fearful thoughts, anxiety-provoking situations, "offending" personalities or events, and anything else that provokes in you stressful, unkind, hostile, or pessimistic thoughts. Note them all casually, and notice the way these thoughts morph into negative emotions that produce a perception of threat.

As you experience each of these negative feelings, don't try to change them. Just observe them, and if you criticize, blame, or condemn yourself for thinking and feeling negatively, simply observe this as another negative thought. As you observe stress-provoking thoughts, tell yourself, *This thought or feeling exists in me, not in reality.* Then take a moment and allow the truth of this to sink in. Don't believe the stressful thought. The reason behind this practice is that if you don't believe an anxious, stressful, pessimistic thought, it will have no power. It will simply be a thought that comes and goes instead of turning into stress, anxiety, or depression.

Once you have done this, tell yourself, *I could see peace instead of this.* Focusing on the idea of a peaceful alternative, and repeating this idea to yourself in an unhurried manner, will help your perception of the world change in a positive way.

Finally, as your attitude shifts, remember that although negative thoughts and feelings are in you, they are not you. They come and go like clouds. But the essence of your being is like the blue sky these clouds travel through and sometimes cover. Let your mind go completely and become the blue sky for a moment.

Practice the Thought Awareness Tool every day, throughout the day, until it becomes your immediate response to stress-provoking thoughts and perceptions. You will find the step-by-step process for using this tool at the end of the chapter, along with the link for downloading a copy of it.

As you practice this process, your lower brain will begin to quiet down. Most of our stressful, anxious thoughts happen unconsciously, outside of our awareness. Until these thoughts are made conscious, they will continue to automatically trigger the stress response system. But as the lower brain begins to receive the message from you that this or that thought is just a thought, not an emergency, and that there is nothing to fear, it will begin to stand down. This will not only preserve the energy that stressful thinking drains, but it will prevent you from acting on a paranoid thought and misperception in a way you'll later regret.

If your day is particularly busy or stressful, you can use a shorter application of this tool. Whenever a fearful thought begins to make inroads into your emotional well-being in the form of depression, anxiety, or worry, intervene by simply by taking a deep breath, letting your mind go for a moment, and then silently stating, "I can replace this feeling of [depression, anxiety, or worry] with peace." Keep repeating the idea until you feel some sense of relief.

The key to using the Thought Awareness Tool effectively is using it repeatedly. At first, it might feel awkward or difficult to apply, and even hard to remember to do it, but stick with it. The more you practice it, the easier it becomes to do and the more it works. Eventually it changes your brain's autopilot from one that habituates stress to one that keeps you at peace.

The following examples reveal the enormous difference the Thought Awareness Tool can make. These examples present two people with very different problems, but who stress about their particular problem in the same way.

The first example is of a man whose wife recently died after a long illness. In his grief, he ruminates over things he thought he could have and should have done for her, and these thoughts eventually morph into the fear that he's failed her. He thinks he should have quit work and stayed home with her in the last few months of her life, forgetting that doing so would have run the risk of losing his health insurance. He mulls over his wife's last few days, as she went in and out of consciousness. He feels there might have been something more he could have done to help her survive the crisis. All of this recrimination snowballs into a litany of mistakes he perceives he's made over their thirty-year marriage, culminating in his judgment that he was not the good husband he'd once believed himself to be. This initial reaction is common for people who've lost a loved one.

The second example is something that happens every day in business. It's the shock that senior managers feel when the company loses a major client, causing a significant loss of revenue. Of course, this represents a real crisis that requires clear thinking, but initially the crisis can overwhelm leaders. At first they become angry and often point the finger at other people, but soon they find their own finger pointing back at them. They can become frightened by all the mistakes their fear says they must have made. "The buck stops with me," a leader usually says, "so I must have failed in some way." This turns into the fear of having failed everyone from investors to employees to their family. Their emotional overwhelm completely discounts the fact that for years, they have led a successful division that provided exciting jobs and a good living for scores of people. They are smart enough to deal with the situation, and know that they have to quickly come up with a plan and rally the troops, but their present state of mind immobilizes them.

Both of these people in the examples had allowed their fear to dominate their attitude and cause them to think negatively about themselves. This self-condemnation makes a difficult situation worse. The downturn in attitude in both examples is a result of believing thoughts that are fundamentally untrue. When fear grips the mind, it becomes difficult to see how simply eliminating fearful thoughts can instantly make everything better, including higher-brain function. The prescription is to begin monitoring painful, stress-provoking thoughts and observe how much of one's painful emotional state is a product of thoughts, not reality. The next step is to refute stressful thoughts simply by refusing to believe any of them. Accomplishing this is a matter of going past whatever the negative ego says until one reaches the refreshing, elevating experience on the other side of not believing the painful picture fear paints. What naturally emerges is a calmer, more intelligent, more realistic and optimistic way of seeing and being that opens the way to moving forward. In the example of a grieving husband, once the way forward becomes clear, the husband is free to grieve his loss while holding in his heart the dignity of the love he and his wife shared; in the example of the company losing a client, the senior manager was free to look at the company's problem fearlessly and to inspire the management team to fix it.

Your Practice This Week

- Download the document called "Attributes of a Dynamically Peaceful Attitude," print it, and then check off the three qualities you want to accentuate in the coming week. Post this list at home and at work where you will notice it often.

- Every day look at the three items you selected from the list that you want to accentuate and find ways to do so.
- Use the Thought Awareness Tool during the coming week, each day, all day long. At times, doing this process may feel unpleasant; don't let this stop you from continuing. At other times, you might judge yourself critically for the amount of negative thinking you're uncovering. This might even make you feel discouraged or hopeless. Simply observe these judgments and feelings as more of the same anxious, stress-provoking thoughts you are actively bringing into awareness.

And Keep Practicing the Following

- Continue starting your day in quiet. Make it as important as having your morning cup of coffee or tea (that is, if you drink coffee or tea).

Tools

Thought Awareness: *I could see peace instead of this.* Read this page each day, until you are clear on how to apply this process.

- Be aware of stressful, fearful thoughts, anxiety-provoking situations, "offending" personalities or events, or anything else that provokes in you stressful, unkind, hostile, or pessimistic thoughts. Note them all casually, whenever they occur. Notice the way these thoughts morph into negative emotions that produce a perception of threat.
- Initially, as you look at a negative thought or feeling, don't try to change it. Simply observe it. If you criticize, blame, or condemn yourself for thinking and feeling negatively, simply observe this as another negative thought.

- Tell yourself, *This thought or feeling is in me, not in reality.* Take a moment and see the truth in this. Let it sink in.
- Don't believe a stressful thought. If you don't believe an anxious, stressful, pessimistic thought, it has no power. It's just a thought that comes and goes. When you don't believe a negative thought, it doesn't turn into stress, anxiety, or depression.
- Tell yourself, *I could see peace instead of this.* Repeat this idea to yourself in an unhurried manner as you watch your perception of the world change.
- Conclude by remembering that although negative thoughts and feelings are in you, they are not you. They come and go like clouds. But the essence of your being is like the blue sky these clouds travel through and sometimes cover. Let your mind go completely and become the blue sky for a moment.

4

The Question at the Bottom of Stress

Initially, as people begin to work with the Thought Awareness Tool and uncover the negative, stress-provoking thoughts their brains generate, they usually run into thoughts that are difficult to escape. They often ask me, "What if this fear is real—what if it's true?" I tell them it's important to challenge the thought to see whether their anxiety is about a serious threat that actually exists or just some fear thinking up catastrophes. If we give in to fear, things are likely to escalate into a strong stress reaction, releasing a flood of stress hormones that can rob us of the brainpower we need to solve the problem. There is a process that helps you investigate a fearful perception before it takes you on a long walk off a short pier. It's called the What Am I Afraid Of? Tool. You will find the step-by-step process for using this tool at the end of the chapter, along with the link to an audio file in which I guide you through the process.

This tool invites you to deconstruct a situation that troubles you by repeatedly asking yourself to consider the question "What am I afraid of?" For example, you might be afraid that you don't have enough money for your vacation. You then take that answer and turn it into the next question, asking yourself, "If this fear were actually true, then what would I be afraid of?" Your answer to that might be that everyone in your family will blame and hate you. Again, you take this answer and turn it into the next question, repeating the process until you've taken it as far it goes, which is usually five or six rounds.

In using the What Am I Afraid Of? Tool, it is very important to allow the language of the lower, primitive brain to speak without editing or sugarcoating its words. The lower brain speaks in raw and often catastrophic terms. It's not interested in facts. It's interested in survival and often jumps to crazy, fearful conclusions. Your job is to let it speak so you can get to the bottom of the nightmare the lower brain sees and to which it's reacting.

Once your list is complete, read each statement, removing the preface *I'm afraid* and turning each one into a factual statement. For example, instead of saying "I'm afraid I don't have enough money for our vacation," you would read it as a fact: "I don't have enough money for our vacation." Instead of saying "I'm afraid everyone in my family will hate me," you would read it as "Everyone in my family will hate me." You read all the statements to yourself in this way as if you are telling a story.

The last step is to put each and every statement to the test by asking whether it's true. In the case of this example, you would ask if it's really true that there is no way to come up with money for the vacation. Is it really true that if you disappoint your family they'll hate you? And so on.

The best way to show you how this process works is to tell you a story about a sales executive I'll refer to as Justin. Although the story is fictitious, it's typical of how the process unfolds.

Justin has been working on a sale for almost a year that, had he landed it, not only would have met his sales quota ahead of schedule but would also have earned him a bonus. Sadly, just when the sale was about to close, a gatekeeper in the prospective company derailed it, based on what Justin perceived as this person's fear that the product would make part of his function obsolete. Everything stalled, and Justin was afraid the deal was dead, which distressed him to no end. For the better part of three weeks, his thoughts produced an emotional state that fluctuated between anger, fear, and discouragement, and he was sinking into depression. He reached the point where he couldn't come up with a creative approach to the problem, and he was afraid he was losing his competitive drive. So Justin makes an appointment with me, and I take him through the What Am I Afraid Of? process.

I begin by asking Justin, "In this situation, what are you afraid of?"

"That the sale is dead," is his answer.

"What are you afraid of if you lose the sale?" I ask.

"Everything I've worked for this last year won't come to anything," he says. "It means I let everyone down, and it makes it harder for me to make my sales quota."

"What's the fear of not making your quota?"

He answers, "Well, my company will start thinking about letting me go and getting someone who can close a deal."

"And what's the fear of getting fired?" I ask.

"I'll end up broke and lose my home and fail my wife," he says.

"And what's the fear in losing your home and failing your wife?"

"It means I failed at life," he replies.

"And what's the fear of failing at life?" I ask.

"No one will respect me," Justin says. His face turns ashen and he drops his head. When I ask him to describe what he's feeling, he says, "I feel completely worthless, like the complete loser my father said I'd become." You can see in this answer how deeply rooted our fears can be.

"And what's the fear of failing everyone and no one respecting you?"

"I'll end up living under a bridge, with no one who cares about me," he says. Then he laughs, although he looks upset. It is a ridiculous statement to make, but it isn't his logical mind that is speaking, it's his lower brain.

In the next phase of the process, I turn his fear-based responses into a narrative that I recite to Justin. "The story you're telling yourself is that you're going to lose this sale, and everything you've been working toward for the last year will have amounted to nothing. Your company will fire you and replace you with someone better. You'll end up broke and lose your home. You'll have failed your wife. No one who matters to you will ever respect you again because you're a loser, just like your father said. And you're going to end up homeless and forsaken."

This is the story that has been running in the back of Justin's mind for the last three weeks, tyrannizing him and exciting an array of upsetting emotions. Think back to what I said in chapter 1 about "contextual fear conditioning." It refers to the way the lower brain associates something in the present situation with an upset from the past that the brain stored in its emotional memory. Contextual fear conditioning causes us to perceive a threat in a situation that isn't actually there. For Justin, the failure he perceived in the spoiled sale reactivated the trauma of his father's condemnation. To the lower brain, his father's rejection portends the day when Justin will be thrown out on the street and forsaken, which is the lower brain's deepest fear. Believing a story like the one projected onto the screen of Justin's mind would stress and frighten anybody. Some people might commiserate with Justin, thinking, *The poor man. I hope he finds a way to secure the sale so his life isn't ruined.* Some people might become anxious if his story strikes a nerve. Others might look at Justin with disgust, as if they thought he really was a loser. The one thing all these reactions would share in common is that, to some degree, they believe Justin's story.

In the next part of the process, I conduct an inquiry to see if any of Justin's statements are true. Having read this far in this book, you now know how destructive stress hormones are to higher-brain function. They're neurotoxic, which means they lock us into fight, flight, or freeze, where all we see is a problem with no solution. Thus it's critical to determine whether our fears are valid before allowing events to proceed to the next stage of stress, which will flood the brain with toxic stress hormones. So I guide Justin through an inquiry to separate fact from fiction. I begin by asking, "Have you lost the sale entirely?"

"Well," Justin says, "maybe not entirely. I could resurrect it, but it's politically tricky. I'd have to go over the head of the gatekeeper."

"So if you could figure out an effective way to do that, it means it's not over yet. Right?" I ask.

"Yes, I suppose so," he answers. "If I could figure that out, it could give the sale another chance." Justin goes on to say that his boss is politically savvy about getting around touchy issues, but Justin has been avoiding his boss. He didn't want to tell him that the sale was in deep trouble until he had a plan to fix it. And, of course, he hasn't been able to come up with a decent plan because he is too distressed to think creatively. Then, all at once, it dawns on him that his fear has trapped him in a kind of catch-22, preventing him from asking his boss to help with a political strategy, which was the only plan he really needed. This revelation makes him smile, and for the first time he relaxes back into the chair.

Next I ask, "If you can't resurrect the sale, does it really mean everything you've worked on this last year adds up to nothing?"

"Well, it's actually not a total loss," he answers. "I developed better collaterals for our product and refined a PowerPoint presentation that's much better than the old one. Other people on the sales team have even begun using the materials in their sales presentations."

"Well, that must feel like an accomplishment," I say.

"Yes, actually, it does," Justin says. "My boss gave me kudos for it."

"Do you really think it's possible your boss might fire you if you don't make this sale?"

"No," he answered. "I have other irons in the fire. If I can refocus, I can make my numbers."

"And what about your wife and your friends? Do you really believe they don't love you unconditionally?"

"No, of course not," he says.

Finally, I ask Justin if he thinks it might be time to get help with forgiving his father so he can let go of the fear of ending up a loser. He says he is willing to do that. Then I hand Justin the list of fear statements he made and ask, "Who would you be without these fearful thoughts?"

"I'd be a lot calmer and a lot smarter," he says. "And I'd be a lot happier at the end of the day when I come home to my wife."

The fearful stories we tell ourselves when we're stressed or afraid are generated by the lower brain. The lower brain always speaks in these raw, disturbing terms. It's in survival mode, and what it sees is a bad dream. The lower brain was using Justin. The realistic account that emerged when these fears were dispelled sent Justin on his way to using his higher brain to function at the top of his game. And the realistic account is always more sensible, more upbeat, more optimistic and forward moving. Awareness makes the situation conscious. Now our conscious mind can see the choice that is always before us, which boils down to empowering either fear or peace.

Justin's story had a happy ending. When he went back to work on the sale, he was in top form. Stress no longer undermined his effort to close the deal.

Now I invite you do this process. You can begin right now by asking yourself what you're currently afraid of. Reflect on this question for a moment. Write it down and process it by doing the What Am I Afraid Of? exercise.

Your Practice This Week

Once this week, perform the What Am I Afraid Of? Tool, using the fear you identified.

And Keep Practicing the Following

- Continue using the Thought Awareness Tool.
- Continue using the Starting the Day in Quiet Tool.

Tools

What Am I Afraid Of?

- Ask yourself, *What am I afraid of at present?* Drop into this anxious, unsettling space and sit with this question. When you have your answer, write it down at the very top of a piece of paper.
- Draw a line down the middle of the paper. At the top of the left column write: *What am I afraid of?* At the top of the right column write: *Inquiring if it's true.*
- Take your initial fear and turn it into the next question. Ask yourself, *If this fear at the top of the page is true, what am I afraid of?* Record your answer in the left column.
- Turn that fear into the next question. *And if this fear I just recorded were true, what am I afraid of?* Record it.
- Repeat this sequence three of four more times or until you sense you have reached the bottom of your anxiety about this situation.

The What Am I Afraid Of? Audio Story:
A seven-and-a-half-minute audio in which Don describes how the What Am I Afraid Of? process works and why to use this tool.

http://www.beyondword.com/theendofstress/tag2_What-Am-I
-Afraid-Of-Part-1-The-Story.mp3

What Am I Afraid Of? Audio Walkthrough, part 2:
A nine-and-a-half-minute audio in which Don steps you through the What Am I Afraid Of? process to address a fear you have.

http://www.beyondword.com/theendofstress/tag3_What-Am
-I-Afraid-Of-Part-2-The-Process.mp3

Conducting the Inquiry

- Look at each of your fears, one at a time. Ask, "Am I 100 percent certain this statement is true?"
- What statement is more realistic? Record that statement in the right-hand column.
- Go through your list of fears, repeating the above two steps for each of your fears.
- Next, read the What Am I Afraid Of? column as if you are reading a story. How does that feel? Then read the Inquiring if It's True column, again as if telling a story. How does that feel? Which did you choose to believe when stressed?
- Finally, ask yourself, "Who would I be without these fears?" Write your answer down on the back of the paper.

GETTING TO CHOICE

The Mind-Set That Transforms Your Brain

5

Practice Makes Perfect

It takes a simple but consistent practice to produce the positive neuroplasticity that enables the brain to function fully. So before venturing further, I want to devote this chapter to discussing the importance of practice, starting with a story about an extremely stressed woman who experienced a breakthrough while using the tools this book provides. It illustrates what can happen when you practice every day.

A woman I'll call Lilah really had her hands full. She was a single mother of two, the primary caregiver for her elderly father, and a project manager in a high-pressure start-up company. She was quite stressed. The holidays were the straw that broke the camel's back, and she was rushed to the emergency room with heart palpitations. Her visit to the ER turned out to be a wake-up call instead of a heart attack, motivating her to do something about stress. A friend of hers, who'd attended one of my seminars, sent her the Starting Your Day in Quiet Tool and the Thought Awareness Tool. For three weeks, Lilah followed the plan, waking up twenty minutes earlier each morning to start her day in quiet, practicing gratitude, and framing her day by evoking a positive, dynamically peaceful attitude. During the day,

she diligently practiced the Thought Awareness Tool and was flab-
bergasted by the number of stressful thoughts and judgments that
her brain was generating throughout the day. Because she was practicing, she became increasingly aware of the way negative thoughts
quickly morph into upsetting emotions. She began to see how, at
times, these upsets caused her to misperceive situations and jump to
rather drastic conclusions, placing her in conflict with whomever or
whatever was involved. What surprised her most was how many of
the stressful thoughts she uncovered had been occurring habitually,
outside of her awareness, operating in the background in ways that
darkened the foreground. By the end of the first week, Lilah came to
realize that the level of negative thinking she was habitually running
could not help but produce a stressful day. She could see that even
her fatigue had more to do with the emotional reactions that stressful
thoughts and judgments produced than with the day's circumstances.

At first, when Lilah detected a stress-provoking thought, she
reacted by judging herself. *I'll never change,* she'd think, followed by,
If I don't change, I'm going to die of a heart attack. But she quickly
realized that self-doubts were just more stress-provoking thoughts.
As she practiced not judging the negative content but simply observing it, she noticed that her reactivity gradually began to quiet down.
Soon she was laughing at her stressful thoughts; what had once been
a horror movie was now a sitcom. As she worked at not believing
her stressful thoughts and perceptions, she began to experience the
freedom on the other side of fear. It was something of a revelation
for her when she recognized that being stress free had more to do
with managing her thoughts than controlling people or manipulat-
ing circumstances.

She began to notice that many of the people around her were
stressed but she wasn't—at least not as much as before. Something
inside of her had quieted down. She said it was like choosing not to
drink at a cocktail party and discovering how altered drinkers become.

Then came a breakthrough. One day, after three weeks of practicing the tools, Lilah was walking to her car across the company parking lot, and for no reason she could identify, she experienced a spontaneous moment of joy. She stopped and stood still for a moment, and as she looked around, she thought, *What a beautiful world.* She described it as a "perfect moment."

It's ironic that what clears the space for that perfect moment is our willingness to spend some time observing all the imperfections that stressful thoughts perceive.

Joy is what we feel when we've been liberated from stressful, worried, and anxious thinking. In that moment we know what it means to live without fear and stress. That's mind changing. It's life changing.

So far, you've been working on becoming more keenly aware of the experience you don't want—meaning stress. From this point forward, you'll be working with tools and processes that offer the experience you do want. It all comes back to practice. Through practice, you are building the brain structure to change stress to ease, fear to peace, powerlessness to power. As I said in chapter 1, practice takes discipline, and discipline is simply remembering what you want and then choosing it consistently. As I've mentioned already, the reward is doing well and being well, on your way to flourishing. What could be more deserving of your effort and intent than a result that gives you this? And what could be more motivating than getting what you want?

At first the process of change may seem frustrating. You may find that you quickly fall back into an old routine, or that your busy life is blocking you from making the time to practice the exercises the book has assigned. You might even feel guilty about it or think that you are not good enough or disciplined enough to make a meaningful change. As you now know, the prescription for that kind of negative thinking is to run it through the Thought Awareness Tool to dispel it. You can make this change. The key, as with anything you're trying to achieve, is to not give up. Try and try again until you achieve the momentum that can carry you to your goal.

I often hear people say that it's hard to choose peace in this hectic world. But when you reflect on it, it becomes clear that stress and fear are what make life hard. A dynamically peaceful approach makes everything easier, whether it's doing the laundry and mowing the lawn or pursuing your career and raising your family. The more you practice peace, the easier it gets. Neurologically, practice wires the algorithm for a new behavior or brain state into a part of your brain called the basal ganglia. It's the place where the brain stores the cues, patterns, and rewards that form your habits. Through practice, you program the pattern that cues the reward of peace when a stressor raises its head. But you can't know the reward peace bestows until you practice being at peace.

There is a famous experiment that illustrates how this autopilot works.[1] Researchers at MIT had discovered that an animal with a damaged basal ganglia struggled with learning new routines. The researchers wanted to see if the basal ganglia might be involved in forming and changing habits, so they wired up the brains of lab rats in order to discern what was happening in their tiny heads, placed the critters in a T-shaped maze, and hid an enticing piece of chocolate at the farthest corner of the maze. The first few times the rats were placed in the maze, they seemed to smell the chocolate but were unable to locate it. As they sniffed, scratched, and milled around, the data showed that their brains were working overtime to find the chocolate. Gradually, through trial and error, the rats figured out where it was. After that, they routinely made a beeline straight for the reward at the far corner of the maze without the perplexing struggle of having to figure things out. The surprising thing the researchers discovered from the brain data was that as each rat learned the way to the chocolate, mental activity decreased. Even activity in memory centers quieted down. The brain became quiet. The algorithm had taken over and was running like an autopilot. No more hard work. The process of trial and error culminating in the reward had wired the change into the rat's basal ganglia.

So, here's the message: practice the tools and processes in this book. They will get you to the chocolate faster. But if you wake up on the wrong side of the bed or get caught in a stress reaction, don't judge yourself. Let it go. Life is a trial-and-error process we all go through on our way to reaching higher plateaus. The old maxim "practice makes perfect" isn't about you being perfect; it's about progressing toward excelling at life.

The practice of inner peace strengthens your capacity to face difficulty without being afraid of it. It's the inner strength that remains calm, clear, and creative when you face a difficult situation. But achieving peace doesn't mean you will never again experience anger, agitation, or anxiety, or that you will never again confront stressors. There will also be times when you'll be pulled into a storm of stress, staggered by bad news, or caught in the grip of your own emotional negativity. Something Ralph Waldo Emerson said can help you let go of a less-than-perfect day. Emerson wrote,

> Finish each day and be done with it. You have done what you could. Some blunders and absurdities no doubt crept in; forget them as soon as you can. Tomorrow is a new day; begin it well and serenely and with too high a spirit to be encumbered with your old nonsense. This day is all that is good and fair. It is too dear, with its hopes and invitations, to waste a moment on yesterdays.[2]

I've framed Emerson's statement and placed it on my desk. At the close of the day, just before I leave the office, I look at it to remind myself to let the day go and "be done with it." I imagine tomorrow, "with its hopes and invitations," and I feel the passion in my heart for the purpose I want to fulfill and the dreams I want to achieve. Then I infuse the atmosphere of my office with this joyful feeling so it's there to lift me up when I return in the morning.

If I feel the pain of a blunder I committed during the day, I read Emerson's statement. Sometimes, when I've blundered big, I have to read it two or three times, taking in every word until I completely let go. Reaching that point of letting go is always a great relief. It feels like I've set down a heavy suitcase or taken off a tight shoe, and it allows me to move forward again with ease and high purpose.

Keep Practicing the Following

- Continue using the Thought Awareness Tool.
- Perform the What Am I Afraid Of? exercise if a thought comes up that you have difficulty letting go.
- Continue using the Starting the Day in Quiet Tool.

6

Quietly Engaged, Fully Present

n her book *Operating Instructions*, Anne Lamott quotes one of her friends, who said, "My mind is like a bad neighborhood that I try not to go into alone."[1] This image makes us laugh because we can all relate to the bad neighborhood of our own mind when it becomes pointlessly preoccupied with a stream of incessant, chaotic thinking that judges, criticizes, blames, complains, defends, and attacks, sometimes yelling right out loud with sprays of spit. I'd venture to guess that on a bad day, the streets of this bad neighborhood can fill with thousands of stressful thoughts, and that most are repeat offenders. It can plunge the mind into the dark waters of catastrophic thinking, as it did with Justin, the salesman in the What Am I Afraid Of? exercise.

Think back to the last time when, like Justin, you were overwhelmed by the fear of failing. The thought of failure floods the mind with images of terrible calamities. It drags you from the present moment back into the failures and disappointments of the past, which in turn makes the future seem nightmarish. Your emotions fluctuate between anxiety, anger, and depression until at some point it all escalates into a storm of fear. But most, if not all, of the turbulence is fueled by mind-made illusions. It's how William Shakespeare once described life as "a tale told by an idiot, full of sound and fury, signifying nothing."[2] But Shakespeare also said, "I feel within me a peace above all earthly dignities; a still and quiet conscience."[3]

This "still and quiet conscience" is attained by stepping out of the tight corner that stressful thinking paints us into. How? By letting go of fear and then consciously stepping into the present moment, ready to engage life with a quiet, open, and receptive mind, remembering that now is the only time there is, the only time in which you ever exist. Miss this moment and you miss your life. In the quiet of the present moment, the false image of yourself fades. The image of a threatening world fades. The judgments you project onto other people fade. Your fear of failure fades, and what takes its place is the bold possibility of what you can create right here, right now, when you're not afraid of anything. Can you imagine a state of mind without fearful illusions? Try to remember a time—even one that only lasted a minute, maybe even less—when nothing came to interrupt your peace, when you were certain you were loved and safe, and your future was not in doubt. Remember a specific place or time when you felt this way. Remember how quiet your mind became, how at ease you felt in that setting, how fully present you were.

If you can't remember such a moment, imagine one. Relax into the possibility of being completely at peace and fully present. Make it vivid. Try to picture this moment extending until it becomes a whole day. Now imagine it extending to become your experience *every day*. Your best day, every day. This might give you a hint of what it would be like to be free of the fearful illusions that a brain chronically under stress generates. Without these illusions, there would be no fear, no stress, no doubt, and no attack.

You might think that engaging life and work with a quiet mind that's fully present would mean you wouldn't be motivated to get anything done or have impact in the world. The irony is that being quietly engaged and fully present as you approach whatever you have to manage actually makes you more powerful. It's a quality of presence that flows into whatever you are doing, alleviating stress and making you calmer, more attentive, and more in harmony with other people and conditions.

Gerald Jampolsky, the famous psychiatrist and father of a school of psychology based on attitude, was invited to attend a board of directors meeting of a large corporation. There had been months of disagreement about how to address specific problems in that company, and the disagreement was becoming divisive. Jerry was asked to attend the meeting and consult with the group on how to shift the conflict. Throughout the entire meeting, Jerry simply sat there quietly in a peaceful state of mind, feeling compassion for how stuck the group was. He just listened as people argued among themselves. After the meeting, a number of people came up to Jerry and thanked him for the great things he had said and how much it helped them understand things better. He hadn't said *anything*, yet somehow his quiet presence helped some of the directors see things differently, from a clearer place. The great Irish poet W. B. Yeats asserted that we all are capable of passing into that state of quiet that is the condition of vision:

> Images form themselves in our minds perpetually as if they were reflected in some pool. . . . We can make our minds so like still water that beings gather around us that they may see, it may be, their own images, and so live for a moment with a clearer, perhaps even with a fiercer life because of our quiet.[4]

We have all been touched by the quiet presence of another person. People often say that just being around their grandmothers, for example, helped them feel much more peaceful, as if everything was always all right, even in a difficult situation. They had a way of taking the stress out of a situation. For me that person was my Irish Catholic godmother. She had a face that seemed to shine with light and a way of being that was very calm and dignified. Our home was full of the pandemonium that my two brothers, two sisters, and I could make. But when Genevieve came to visit, we all quieted down and behaved much better. We loved being in her presence. It made the world feel right, and she had a way of making us feel noble, often without saying a word. The quality of her presence communicated love and respect more than words would have.

Quietly engaged, fully present is the very essence of peace. We often assume that we have to strive for peace, but the fact is our brain is already wired for peace. It's part of human nature. The problem is that we don't give peace the chance to flip the switch for a better experience. Instead, stress becomes our autopilot and the day devolves into fight, flight, or freeze. But peace is always right here, waiting for you to simply choose it.

The Thirty-Second Time-Out for Peace Tool

There is a simple, easy tool for flipping the switch to peace, and in just thirty seconds. In fact, the exercise is called the Thirty-Second Time-Out for Peace Tool. Here's how it works: Disengage from whatever you are doing and step away from the world for a moment. Let go of what you are thinking or feeling and relax. Let your mind go, and as you do, allow your brain to relax, the same way a stretched muscle relaxes when you stop flexing it. You might even experience a tingling feeling on the top of your head.

Let your neck and shoulders soften, and as you do, let your mind go even more. Let go of everything for just a moment, and allow the world as you perceive it to fall away. No worries, no problems, no goals, nothing to prove.

Now take a slow, easy breath and, as you exhale, let your mind open wide. Be right here, right now, and allow peace to begin to emerge as your experience, all by itself.

You can perform this short exercise just about anywhere or anytime. You can do it while taking a shower, walking to a meeting, sitting in your car during a traffic jam, waiting for a friend to arrive, or looking out a window on a rainy day. Try it a few times throughout the day. At the end of the chapter, there is a link to download a copy of this tool.

There is a way of applying the Thirty-Second Time-Out for Peace Tool that tests your resolve to be at peace. It comes from an exercise used in treating type-A personalities, which refers to highly strung, highly driven, extremely stressed individuals, who run a much higher risk of developing heart disease. To help type-As avoid an early grave, cardiologist Meyer Friedman designed a set of exercises to challenge them to practice the art of being at peace. One of the more challenging exercises was to choose the longest line during checkout at a store and stand in it, practicing inner peace. I invite you to do this exercise for one week. As you're standing in the longest line, take note of your thinking pattern. Notice any resistance to doing the exercise. Notice any pattern of thinking that says you don't have time—that you need to hurry to the next thing on your to-do list. Become aware of any judgments you're making about how long the clerk is taking, or how somebody is dressed, or about the "junk" in someone's cart. Tell yourself *I could see peace instead of this*, just as you would using the Thought Awareness Tool. Then perform the practice using the Thirty-Second Time-Out for Peace Tool.

The Getting Clear Tool

There is a simple tool based on traditional meditation practices that can deepen your experience of peace even more. Research definitively shows that meditation reduces symptoms of stress and anxiety and can maintain these reductions in patients with stress, generalized anxiety disorder, panic disorder, or even panic disorders with agoraphobia.[5] It moves your mind to a better neighborhood. There is an approach called Getting Clear that can help you get out of that neighborhood. It helps clear your mind of incessant chatter. Practiced daily, this tool gradually expands the space between all those pointless thoughts to eventually reach that wide-open space where peace and quiet reside.

The Getting Clear Tool takes you through a very simple process that only takes a few minutes to complete. The goal is to progressively increase your practice from five minutes to twenty minutes or more. To begin, sit comfortably in a chair, with your feet on the ground and your hands folded and resting on your lap. Close your eyes and follow your breath for a few moments. Then just observe what your mind is thinking, feeling, and imagining, without becoming involved in your thoughts. Refrain from judging them or trying to change them. The task is simply to observe the mental and emotional content in your head. Early in the process, it may seem that there is nothing but chatter and chaos. It may seem that your mind is lost in a proliferation of thoughts, judgments, and evaluations. The task remains the same: simply observe this. The mind will present you with the impulse to do something other than this process. The body will also demand attention. Ignore it.

Toward the end of the five-minute process, you're asked to lay these thoughts, feelings, and imaginings aside, not separately, but all of them as one—they're really all the same—and to allow a deeper, more expanded experience of self to naturally emerge. The quality of mind that is able to observe and slip past all the thinking is not a thought; it is freedom from thought. It is the field that is out beyond the stress and anxiety of a worried mind. It is the very essence of who and what you are.

When your mind is quiet and fully present, you may be pleasantly surprised by how beautiful reality can be. Additionally, the research shows that meditation generates positive neuroplasticity, meaning the more you meditate, the more your brain rewires to maintain a stress-free experience.[6] At the end of the chapter, there is a link to download a copy of this tool, as well as an audio file to guide you in using it.

Marking the Moment

Whatever glimpse you get of peace, either when using the Getting Clear Tool to meditate or whenever any experience opens you up, mark the moment. I think marking these expansive moments is so important that I designed a tool for it, simply called Mark the Moment. That glimpse of peace is golden. We often think the moment didn't last long enough and believe it had no lasting effect or value. We might even judge ourselves as inept and think we're incapable of peace. It's not so. This glimpse of peace and quiet is something important. Let it imprint on your brain. Don't try to hold on to the experience—just enjoy it while it lasts and don't fret when it subsides. When you stop and Mark the Moment in this way, you make it matter. Your brain begins to relate to it as a reward that a routine of mindfulness cued, which wires it as a habit. The next time the experience of peace or joy happens, it is likely to be more vivid and last longer.

Thomas Merton, one of America's great spiritual thinkers, said, "All problems are resolved and everything is clear, simply because what matters is clear."[7] Part of what the Getting Clear Tool makes clear is what doesn't matter, which is all the incessant thinking. The process helps you bring into awareness and lay aside all those pointless, incessant thoughts so you can open to the deeper experience inside you that does matter. You're asked to mark that expansive moment of peace, regardless of how long it lasted, and make it matter by relating to it as important.

The Getting Clear Tool also dovetails with the Thought Awareness Tool. Part of using the Thought Awareness Tool involves reminding yourself that you could *see peace instead of this*, meaning instead of the bad neighborhood the mind can become. Observing all the incessant chatter is the *this* part of it. So when you're stressed and you think, *I could see peace instead of this*, you recall that expansive moment and use it to point yourself in the direction of peace. In this way, what matters is made clear.

If you don't get a glimpse of peace when doing the Getting Clear meditation, keep practicing. Eventually peace will arise of its own accord. The right hemisphere of the brain is wired to generate an experience of peace. Perhaps no one has provided a more compelling account of the brain's deep neural circuits of peace than Dr. Jill Bolte Taylor, a Harvard neuroanatomist. Unfortunately, it came at the price of a stroke. In 1996, Dr. Taylor woke up to what she described as a pounding pain behind her left eye, which she characterizes as feeling like ice cream brain freeze. Soon her body wasn't functioning properly. As the blood swept over the brain's higher thinking centers, she began to lose cognitive functions, and soon she couldn't speak properly. The crisis would later be diagnosed as an aneurysm in the brain's left hemisphere, causing the brain's logical, linear, intellectual, and linguistic functions to fail. As the intense pain finally subsided, she felt her body disconnect from her mind. All brain chatter went silent, and the right brain took charge of her experience entirely. What followed was an experience that bordered on nirvana. In an interview, Dr. Taylor said,

> In that moment my brain chatter went totally silent. Just like someone took a remote control and pushed the mute button. Any stress related to my job, it was gone. I had found a peace inside of

myself that I had not known before. I experienced pure silence inside of my mind. I had joy.[8]

Whenever I read this passage at a seminar or keynote and ask the audience if anyone would like an experience like that, every hand goes up. It took eight years for Taylor to fully recover the use of her left brain. Happily, the peace she found stayed with her. "I can step into the consciousness of my right hemisphere on command," she said.[9] Once Dr. Taylor's left brain was back online, she was able to use her acumen as a scientist to increase our understanding of these deep neural circuits of peace that reside within each of us.

The Clear Button Tool

There is a tool that provides a shortcut to becoming quietly engaged and fully present. It's called the Clear Button Tool. When anxiety-provoking thoughts are about to set off a stress reaction, you have about ninety seconds to intervene. Miss that ninety-second window and you could face a full-blown stress reaction that could take an hour or more to recover from. The Clear Button Tool gets you through that window in time.[10]

Here's how this tool works: Start by imagining there is a button at the center of your palm. This is the Clear Button. Whenever stressful thinking rears its ugly head and you feel it is about to build into a larger reaction, press the Clear Button with the index finger of the opposite hand, and keep pressing it. As you do this, picture that it is sending a signal to your stress response system to quiet down. While still pressing the button, count to three, taking in a slow, deep breath with each count and thinking of each number as a color. The color you choose does not matter. On the third and final exhale, let go of whatever was stressing you and come into the present moment. When you're sure your burgeoning reaction has quieted down, reengage with the situation without fear, confident in the clarity your calm now affords you. At the end of the chapter, there is a link to download a copy of this tool, as well as an audio file to guide you in using it.

The Clear Button Tool dovetails with the Thought Awareness Tool. Practicing the Thought Awareness Tool makes you more and more skillful at identifying anxious, pessimistic thoughts that set off stress reactions and flood your brain with toxic stress hormones. Because of your proficiency, you will be able to use the Clear Button Tool to break the negative pattern before it turns into a reaction. For example, you might receive an email you perceive to be insulting. You can feel your blood beginning to boil. But because you're able to recognize the negative pattern, you can intervene with the Clear Button Tool and pass through the ninety-second window unscathed.

In some situations, you may have to repeat the Clear Button process two or three times to clear a stressful, fearful thought pattern. Keep pushing the button and counting to three and thinking of a color; it will eventually work. Each time you push the button, you reset the clock on the ninety-second window. Practice until you become proficient at using this tool. Although it is simple, it is quite effective. It will eventually give you the capacity to bust stressful thoughts and judgments at the point of inception.

There is a neurological basis for the Clear Button Tool. As I said in chapter 1, the amygdala is the brain's fear center and is in charge of the stress response system. The amygdala is fully developed in a human being by age two. Thus this neural circuit has the intelligence and patience of a two-year-old. That's why an angry or frustrated coworker in the throes of a full-blown stress reaction often resembles a child throwing a tantrum. Every parent knows you don't use logic or reason on two-year-olds when they are about to throw a tantrum—you distract them. Counting to three and thinking of each number as a color is a form of distraction. And here's the benefit: Under extreme stress, we lose cognitive and emotional capacity. As a result, all we perceive are problems that we can't solve. But once we've quieted the amygdala, preventing a massive dump of stress hormones, the higher brain can take charge and deliver the creative insight to solve the problem.

Your Practice This Week

- Practice the Thirty-Second Time-Out for Peace Tool three or four times each day. At least once this week, practice it while standing in the longest line during checkout at a store.
- Perform the Getting Clear Tool meditation every day. Twice a day is even better. It will pay big dividends for the ten minutes you invest.
- Start using the Clear Button Tool, each day, all day long. Begin by practicing it a few times until you get the hang of it. Then apply it to real-life stressors.

And Keep Practicing the Following

- Continue using the Thought Awareness Tool. People often ask me how long they need to do the Thought Awareness process. My answer is the rest of your life. The same goes for the next bullet point.
- Continue starting each day in quiet.

Tools

The Thirty-Second Time-Out for Peace
- Stop whatever you're doing and step away from the world for a moment.
- Let go of what you were thinking and feeling, and allow yourself to relax a little.

- Feel your brain relax, the same way a stretched muscle relaxes when you stop torquing it.
- Relax even more.
- Now, let go of everything. Just for the moment, allow the world as you perceive it to fall away.
- No worries, no problems, no goals, nothing to prove. Just let everything go for a moment.
- Take a slow, easy breath and, as you exhale, let your mind and heart open wide.
- Allow peace to begin to emerge as your experience, all by itself.

The Thirty-Second Time-Out for Peace Guided Process Audio:

A two-and-a-half-minute audio in which Don walks you through the Thirty-Second Time-Out for Peace guided process.

http://www.beyondword.com/theendofstress/tag4_Thirty
-Second-Time-Out-for-Peace.mp3

The Getting Clear Tool: A Short Meditation

Read this page each day until you are clear on how to do the meditation.

- Sit comfortably in a chair with both feet on the ground, your hands folded and resting on your lap. As you settle in, become aware of your breathing. And on the next breath close your eyes.
- All you are asked to do is observe. Simply be with whatever content your mind generates.
- Notice what you are thinking, feeling, and imagining. Don't become involved in the thoughts; don't judge them or try to change them. Simply observe them.
- At first it may seem there is nothing but chatter and chaos. It may seem that your mind is lost in a proliferation of thoughts, judgments, and evaluations. Observe this.

- Notice the thoughts that come and go, the emotions they carry, and the pictures they paint. Stand back from them by simply observing them.

- The mind will present you with the impulse to do something other than this process. Ignore this impulse. Bring your attention to your breathing and simply observe. The body will also demand attention. Ignore it as well, returning your attention to the process of observing.

- Now allow yourself to sink into your mind, letting go of every kind of interference and intrusion by imagining that you are quietly sinking past them. Lay all these thoughts aside, not separately but all of them as one. They are all the same.

- Let go and allow your mind to take its natural course. Observe your passing thoughts without involvement as you quietly slip past them. The quality of mind that is able to observe and slip past all the thinking is not a thought; it is freedom from thought. It comes from beyond the thinking mind. It is the field that is out beyond ideas of right and wrong, out beyond the stress and anxiety of a worried mind. Relax into the feeling of freedom. Feel it expand as you relax into it.

- Sense the light that shines from it. This is the very essence of who and what you are.

- As you open your eyes, be present, right here, right now.

Getting Clear Tool Guided Process Audio:
A ten-and-a-half-minute audio in which Don walks you through the Getting Clear guided process.

http://www.beyondword.com/theendofstress/tag5_Getting
-Clear-Meditation.mp3

The Clear Button Tool
Read this page each day until you are clear on how to do the process.

- Press the center of your palm and keep pressing it.
- Imagine that an electrical signal travels to the brain and begins to quiet things down.
- Next, become aware of your breath. You are going to count to three, thinking of each number as a color. Here's how:
- Take a breath, count "1," and think red.
- Take a second breath, count "2," and think blue.
- Take a third breath, count "3," and think green.
- As you exhale from the third breath, let go of your mind completely. Relax into the present moment. Be right here, right now. Now, as you refocus on the world around you, make the commitment to be at peace as you relate to whatever problems or stressors come next.

 The Clear Button Tool Audio:
A four-and-a-half-minute audio in which Don explains the Clear Button Tool and guides you through the practice step-by-step.

http://www.beyondword.com/theendofstress/tag6_The-Clear -Button.mp3

7

Calm and Clear Inside—Regardless of What's Happening Outside

In his famous poem *"If—,"* Rudyard Kipling writes,

> If you can keep your head when all about you
> Are losing theirs . . . If you can trust yourself when
> all men doubt you . . .
> If you can wait and not be tired by waiting . . .
> [and] meet with Triumph and Disaster
> And treat those two impostors just the same . . .
> [then] Yours is the Earth and everything that's in it.[1]

By "Earth and everything that's in it," I believe Kipling means the health, wealth, and love most of us want. The Earth is yours simply because you don't become a victim of circumstances when all about you the world is making trouble. Your decision to remain calm inside regardless of what's happening outside makes you larger than circumstances. You're able to move through misfortune without it dragging you down, dampening your spirit, or blocking your path. Your calm allows you to look straight into the eyes of adversity, relate to the situation intelligently, and respond to it with skill, creativity, and resilience. You right the ship, reset your course, and keep moving forward.

This quality of calm, when practiced consistently, can eventually grow into an attitude of fearless self-confidence that stress cannot unsettle. It's the attitude that has the best chance of success in an operating room or a cockpit when things start to get out of control or in sports when a game is on the line. It's called the zone of optimal performance. The zone is defined by that quiet sense of control and the absence of tension that overcomes adversity and succeeds. "There is no doubt that the experience is real,"[2] states John Silva of the University of North Carolina. Yet few people seem to actually believe it, and even fewer believe that the quality of our attitude hands us the Earth and everything in it.

In a dire situation, attitude is often the only arrow left in your quiver, when all that you control is the stance you take on the inside as you face the facts on the outside. The outside, which we call the "world," can be defined as circumstances we'll never completely control: the weather, the economy, politics, the environment, mortgage rates, job security, our relatives, and so on. If you were to make a list of everything you don't completely control in your life, it would be long indeed. However, evolution, or the Universe, or whatever name you give to the force that created you, did not leave you powerless. It gave you the capacity to transcend circumstances through the power of attitude. This is what Karl Menninger meant when he said, "Attitudes are more important than facts."[3] An attitude of fearless self-confidence can transform the hard facts of life into the challenge to make your life a masterpiece. In *Tales of Power* by Carlos Castaneda, don Juan states that "a warrior takes everything as a challenge, while an ordinary man takes everything either as a blessing or as a curse."[4] In other words, the ordinary man's fortunes or misfortunes are governed by circumstances. A warrior makes his own fortune by transcending circumstances.

Stress as a Decline in the Power of Attitude

Stress itself can be defined as a decline in the power of attitude. Richard Lazarus, one of the world's leading stress researchers and coauthor of the landmark work *Stress, Appraisal, and Coping*, breaks stress into two components:

1. *The stressor*, which Lazarus defines as any kind of demand or change that life imposes. A stressor can range from a traffic jam or an unpleasant person or another task added to your to-do list to losing your job or your home going into foreclosure.
2. *Stress*, which he defines as your appraisal that you must deal with the demand or change, followed by your perception that the demand overwhelms your resources.[5]

Most people relate to "resources" in worldly terms, such as time, money, equipment, or the support of other people. All of these resources fit that definition of the "world" I just gave. They all represent conditions that you don't completely control. If attitude is the one resource you control completely in every circumstance—and it is—then stress can be defined as losing touch with the power of attitude. The storms of change and shouts of demands can be raging all around you, but a dynamically peaceful attitude has the power to plant you firmly in the eye of the storm. As a result, you are able to act with the intelligence and reason your higher brain naturally generates because it's not encumbered by a flood of stress hormones.

I often ask seminar participants to deconstruct a recent situation that was particularly stressful. I have them make a list of five or six obvious stressors at play in the situation, such as the way people were behaving, time constraints, distractions, systems that didn't work, or a noisy or dimly lit room. One participant described a situation in which she was working from home and on a conference call with her project team. She was anxiously trying to download a document that repeatedly wouldn't open when her housekeeper began vacuuming in the hall outside her office, which set the dog barking. She had to excuse herself from the call to deal with the noise, which took longer than expected because her dog wouldn't come out from where it was hiding. When she returned to the conference call, the discussion was well under way, and she was informed that in her absence, she'd been volunteered for a task she didn't have the time to do. By this point, she was too exasperated to speak up for fear of overreacting, which meant that her emotional state was as bottled up as a pressure cooker. Friends were coming for dinner in another hour, but by the time the call concluded she was so stressed that she didn't have the energy to cook or socialize. These were the elements that formed her list of stressors. Obviously, she didn't have complete control over most of these issues. The only thing she completely controlled was how she related to each problem, which is *attitude*.

Once participants have their list of stressors, I have them rate each item according to the degree of control they perceived they had, from 0 for no control to 1 through 4 for some control to 5 for complete control. Typically, no one assigns complete control to any item on their list, but there are lots of zeroes. Then I ask the group for a show of hands of who listed their attitude as an element in their stressful encounter. It's rare that anyone raises their hand, even though we've discussed the power of attitude in the previous two sessions. It seems people forget too easily the difference their attitude can make, or they simply don't believe it makes a real difference. We become so focused on external factors that the difference a shift in attitude could have made eludes us completely.

At the end of the exercise, I ask people to reflect on how they might have experienced things differently had they focused on remaining *calm and clear inside, regardless of what was happening outside*. Invariably, people say they would have been less affected emotionally, more skillful and creative in relating to the matter at hand, and able to preserve more of their energy.

Fearless self-confidence is the attitude that can make your life your masterpiece, and it's acquired by learning to be calm and clear inside regardless of what is happening outside. Two obstacles stand in the way. The first obstacle is loss of control. The second is overwhelm.

Loss of Control

Life can become intolerable when we lose control of a situation in which outcomes really matter to us. The emotional factor underpinning loss of control is, of course, uncertainty. We ruminate over what might happen and are not clear what to do to regain control. The attitudinal factor underpinning a loss of control is worse. It takes the form of self-defeat stemming from fearful pessimism, which tells us that whatever control we might have is of little or no consequence. In other words, we think we're powerless to do anything about the situation. Actually, with both of these factors, our uncertainty and self-doubt stem from a painful lack of clarity about what we do and don't control. The anxiety of uncertainty activates your stress response system, which has you jumping to conclusions that predict calamity.

The Three Sane Choices Tool

In his book *The Power of Now*, Eckhart Tolle writes that people have only three options when they are presented with a situation that is intolerable: they can change the situation, walk away from it, or accept it.[6] I've formed these three options into a tool I call Three Sane Choices. This tool can help you regain a calming sense of sanity in the middle of an upsetting situation in which you have little influence or control. Moreover, it can prevent the lower brain from wrecking your sanity by saturating your higher brain with a flood of stress hormones. The choices are simple, straightforward, and sometimes easier said than done. But when applied, they quell your anxiety and restore your sense of control—not necessarily over another person or an event, but in terms of yourself and your ability to choose your own way.

Choice #1: You can decide to change the situation, working to shift matters in a constructive direction.

This choice means you haven't given up on the situation. You're willing to work to regain influence over what you want to have happen. Equally, it means you're willing to adjust to conditions as opposed to rigidly pushing your own agenda. For this choice to work, it could mean you have to become less rigid, less defended, and more open, flexible, and creative with the situation you want to change. Often, it requires a willingness to look at the problem with fresh eyes that are open to new information. It might even entail the willingness to look at what might need to change in you, in terms of your attitude and your approach to securing what you want.

Choice #2: You can decide to walk away from the situation.

The second choice is walking away from a situation that has reached an impasse or completely broken down, in order to recover your clarity and emotional balance. Walking away can also mean closing the chapter on a part of your life that no longer serves you. This choice can be painful and hard to face. It may even require the help of a good therapist to work through the fear that has kept you stuck in an unfulfilling situation or unhealthy relationship. The litmus test for walking away is the feeling of peace that resonates in the quiet of your heart when you consider the choice to move on. Then the challenge becomes having faith in your choice and the courage to follow through with it.

Choice #3: You can accept the situation completely, exactly as it is, without anyone or anything needing to change in any way.

The third choice is to surrender, but in the best sense. It might mean that you don't have a better answer to the problem, or that the current situation isn't as bad as it could be, or that you're willing to admit you don't know what's best for another person. Acceptance is total. It means the end of complaining, judging, blaming, or demanding. Acceptance is an inward shift that challenges you, as Gandhi did, to be the change you want to see in the world.

You can practice with this tool right now. Bring to mind a recent situation that was stressful for you. Make it vivid by remembering where you were and who you were with when it occurred. Recall what you were thinking and feeling as you related to the situation.

Now look at the three choices, and consider which one would have felt right to you in that stressful situation. As you imagine applying this choice, notice what happens to your level of stress. With most people, the level of stress decreases. This is because all three of these choices shift your focus from what's happening outside of you, where you have little or no control, to what's happening inside you, where you have a great deal of control. It orients you back to choosing your own way. Your experience is now in your hands, which quiets the inner conflict. This, in turn, quiets the amygdala way down in the lower brain, and a quiet amygdala means no stress reaction.

These three choices are applicable to nearly any situation, including (and especially) family situations. A friend used this tool to help work through a conflict she felt with her husband. She wanted her husband to connect more with her at the end of the day instead of what he usually did, which was to grab a beer and watch baseball.

Obviously her first choice was to *change the situation*, meaning his behavior. The husband tried to acquiesce, but it didn't amount to much more than a modest check-in, usually by the refrigerator, before he retrieved his beer and headed for the TV. Of course, this wasn't the change she'd envisioned. She became resentful and withdrawn and began to consider the second choice, which was walking away from the relationship. It didn't take long for her to see that walking away wasn't really a serious consideration. It had more to do with bluster from her anger and resentment toward her husband than with what she was actually willing to do.

However, simply looking at this choice helped her realize how much she loved him, which calmed her emotional reactions. She looked back at Choice #1 (changing the situation) and decided that what needed to change, at least for the time being, was her own anger that made her husband wrong. She let that go, took her focus off of her husband, and stopped ruminating over what he was or wasn't doing. Instead, she centered herself on being happy and accepting her husband as he was: beer, baseball, and all. Shifting from a preoccupation with what was happening outside of her to what was happening inside resurrected her sense of self-control and restored her sanity. She could see more clearly the choice between peace and fear, which meant she could be proactive instead of reactive, and that calmed her even more.

Eventually, she joined her husband on the couch, and he taught her all about baseball. She became a big fan, and they even went to games at the ballpark together. It was a level of sharing and intimacy she hadn't expected, which in the end satisfied her original desire.

These three choices are not necessarily fixed decisions; they can also be seen as a process. For example, you may try to change a situation, then find that you're up against another person's resistance to change. So you make the choice to stop banging your head against the wall and accept the person as is. Your reward is inner peace.

Later, if the situation gets worse, you may decide to walk away, or, if the other person's attitude changes, you may again decide to work for change. Your choice can fluctuate as the situation changes or as you change your mind.

Another benefit of this tool is the self-reflection it can facilitate. Imagine a situation that has been difficult for you for a long time and where there is little hope of things changing. It might be about a job or a relationship. When you look at the three choices, your rational mind tells you it's time to move on. Yet despite the clarity, there is another part of you that's insecure or even frightened about making this choice. This leaves you feeling confused and inadequate, or maybe even cowardly. When you look back at the three choices, you now realize the relevant choice at the moment is accepting yourself as stuck. You might consider counseling to help you understand the forces at play within you, which means the decision has shifted to changing the situation, not on the outside, but inside you. If you take that step, by definition you are no longer stuck.

Overwhelm

The second obstacle to becoming calm and clear inside, regardless of what's happening outside, is *overwhelm*. Overwhelm can be defined as the pursuit of multiple external goals without a clear inner purpose. We can become so consumed by our life plan and its long to-do list that we lose all connection to life. Life becomes the insane burden of a thousand things to do. We're prone to become overly concerned with the future, pursuing things we think we need and don't have instead of appreciating what we do have at this moment, right now, where our life is actually happening.

This is not to say that external goals are unimportant. Of course they are. They put a roof over our head, money in our pocket, and food on our table, and once our basic needs are met, they help improve our lot in life. In addition, external goals stretch us to real-ize more of our innate potential. But if our state of mind is governed by the ups and downs of external goals, our life becomes an emo-tional merry-go-round. We often mistakenly believe that achieving an external goal will give us peace and make us happy, but it is not in the nature of external goals to give peace or happiness, at least not to the degree that matters. Temporarily, achieving the goal may provide a sense of elation, accomplishment, or relief, but not lasting peace or happiness. Soon the elation fades into the shadows of the next prob-lem the world imposes. Moreover, research has found that only about 10 percent of our happiness stems from changes in our life situation, meaning we only get a 10 percent lift if we transition from poor to rich, or move from a smaller to a bigger house, or get promoted, or even find our soul mate.[7] On the other hand, 40 percent of our happi-ness rises or falls depending on the quality of our mental state. That's the place to make the investment if happiness matters to you.[8]

Peace, happiness, and joy come from within, not from the world. They are not a thing the world gives or takes away. They are a state of mind we choose, regardless of circumstances. The world is just too unfair and too mercurial to trust with our consciousness. The person you want to be, the life you wish to lead, the purpose you long to fulfill, are too important to leave to chance. They require a clear inner purpose that you put first as you work for the Good Life. The irony is that when a clear inner purpose becomes your primary goal, all your other goals have a way of working out.

So, to summarize, the things you want to achieve in the world represent your external goals. The qualities you want to accentuate within yourself as you pursue external goals represent your inner purpose. The outcome is holistic; it's a happier, more peaceful human being working toward a better situation. The challenge is to get clear about your inner purpose and put it first, so that the way you want to be flows easily into whatever you need to do to get ahead.

The simplest way I've found to infuse a clear inner purpose with external goals is to integrate your to-*be* list into your to-*do* list. There is a form at the end of this chapter for doing exactly this. It's called My To-Be List for My To-Do List. You list in one column the external goals you want to achieve in three areas of your life: business, family, and health. This is your to-do list. Next, you list qualities you want to succeed in being as you work toward the external goals you listed, using the qualities from Attributes of a Dynamically Peaceful Attitude, which is also provided at the back of this chapter. You can assign more than one quality to an external goal; this is your To-Be List. When you've completed the worksheet, post it where you will see it, as a reminder of how you want to be as you work to accomplish your goals.

Commit to looking at the worksheet often during the day. As you do, imagine how you might apply the qualities you want to accentuate. For example, if you want to be more open-minded, receptive, and accepting of other people, imagine yourself listening better and judging less as you work with others. Expect the desired change to happen. Expectancy is why placebos work. Expectancy will also propel your inner purpose to the forefront of your day. The more you focus your attention on the quality you want to change or accentuate, the stronger that quality will become, until eventually it becomes your autopilot. This is not to say you won't fail at times, but don't let failure stop you. Choose again how you want to be. Success is guaranteed if you don't quit.

A Word on Multitasking

Another way we become overwhelmed is multitasking. The "smart" technologies of the twenty-first century have us believing that we can actually juggle ten balls at once, but doing so can lead to overwhelm. We think we're great multitaskers, able to talk on the phone while we're proofing a document, checking a text message, and sending an email. But there is, at best, a two-task limit on what the human brain can handle.[9] We've all experienced those moments when the brain loses track of all the tasks it's trying to accomplish at once. Suddenly you don't know where you are now, where you were last, and where you need to go next. Those moments can set off the stress response system, which means you're likely to freeze up or blow up.

Researchers at Stanford University found that multitasking may even impair cognitive control.[10] Anthony Wagner, one of the researchers in this study, said, "When you're in situations where there are multiple sources of information coming from the external world or emerging out of memory, you're not able to filter out what's not relevant to your current goal. That failure to filter means you're slowed down by that irrelevant information."[11] In one study, multi-taskers were found to take 40 percent longer to get something done.[12] Another study even found that drivers talking on cell phones took longer to reach their destinations.[13] Multitaskers also make twice as many errors[14] and are more stressed[15] than people who don't multi-task. And stress, as you now know, means a loss of the brainpower required to get things done, and to get them done well.

I've found that the best thing to do when you find that multi-tasking is getting out of hand is to first stop everything you're doing. Take a deep breath and follow your breathing for a moment. Be present, here and now, and let your mind relax. If you're still feeling overwhelmed, consider going for a walk. Once you are feeling calm and ready to go back to work, make a list of everything you were try-ing to do and select just one item to focus on. Focus on completing that one task with the aim of doing it well.

Speed Bumps

Let's cover one last thing before closing the discussion on over-whelm. It's about a simple shift in mind-set that can transform an irritating moment, which I call a speed bump, into a gentle tap on the shoulder that reminds you to choose peace.

Speed bumps are those annoying disturbances that happen when you need to concentrate or when you're under pressure to get something done. It's someone at your door interrupting you with a problem when you're working to meet a deadline. It's a printer that stops printing. It's a warning light on your car's dashboard that says you're running out of gas when you're late for a meeting. It's noticing a stain on your clothes just before you're about to make a presentation.

I invite you to practice calling these annoyances speed bumps. For example, if an unavoidable interruption happens, wait for the wave of aggravation to pass and then simply say to yourself, *Speed bump*. Use the phrase as a reminder to stop and smell the roses for a few seconds. Tell yourself, *I could see peace instead of this*. Take a breath, become present, and laugh at the human comedy we are all living though. Then relax for a moment, wake up to the present, and remember that your inner purpose is peace.

Your Practice This Week

- Use the Three Sane Choices Tool to help you regain control of circumstances in which you feel powerless.
- Fill out the My To-Be List for My To-Do List form on page 95. You can also download a printable version of the exercise at theend ofstressbook.com. Once you've completed the worksheet, be sure to post it where you will see it.
- Use the multitasking process on pages 96–99 to break the habit.

And Keep Practicing the Following

- Practice the Thirty-Second Time-Out for Peace Tool three or four times each day.

- Continue using the Getting Clear Tool once every day (twice a day is even better).
- Use the Clear Button Tool to clear a stress-provoking pattern of thinking.
- Continue using the Thought Awareness Tool.
- Continue Starting the Day in Quiet.

Tools

The Three Sane Choices

- Decide to change the situation
- Walk away from the situation
- Accept the situation completely

Three Sane Choices Tool Audio:
A two-and-a-half-minute audio in which Don describes the Three Sane Choices Tool and how to apply it to your life.

http://www.beyondword.com/theendofstress/tag7_Three-Sane-Choices.mp3

My To-Be List for My To-Do List

Instructions

1. First, list in the right-hand column the external goals you want to achieve in each of the categories: business, family, and health.
2. Next, define qualities you want to succeed in being as you work to achieve these external goals, using the list of qualities from the Attributes of a Dynamically Peaceful Attitude exercise shown below. Enter those qualities in the left column. You can use any quality more than once.
3. Then post the worksheet where you will see it, to remind you of *how you want to be* as you do what you have to do.

   *See the following sample or download a printable version

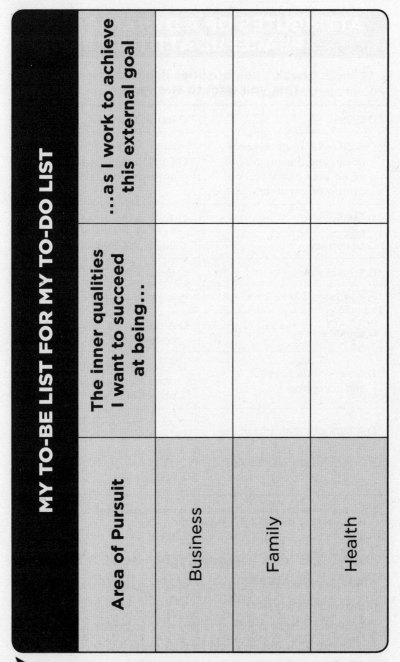

MY TO-BE LIST FOR MY TO-DO LIST		
Area of Pursuit	The inner qualities I want to succeed at being…	…as I work to achieve this external goal
Business		
Family		
Health		

↖ This worksheet is available for download at theendofstressbook.com/worksheets.

ATTRIBUTES OF A DYNAMICALLY PEACEFUL ATTITUDE[16]

Check three qualities listed below that you want to strengthen.

O Calm	O Resilient
O A clear sense of personal power and the integrity to assert your power without overpowering others	O Faith in the face of adversity
O Unafraid	O Trust in the process
O Unhurried	O Joy in the challenge
O Free of worry	O Empathic
O Self-confident	O A willingness to forgive
O Creative	O A disinterest in judging or condemning
O Open-minded, receptive, and accepting	O A felt connection with one's own heart, with others, and with life itself
O A curiosity that is fully present	O An enduring sense of the whole that transcends the fragments
O Energetic	O A sense of the sacred

➤ **This worksheet is available for download at theendofstressbook.com/worksheets.**

Multitasking

- When you find that multitasking is getting out of hand, stop everything you're doing.
- Take a deep breath and then follow your breathing for a moment. Be present, here and now, and let your mind relax.

- If you are feeling overwhelmed, take a break from it all and go for a walk. It can help dispel the stress hormones and refresh your brain.
- When you are ready to go back to work, write down the several things you were trying to do at once. Focus on one task, starting out slow and easy, with the aim of doing it well.

8

Hawaiianizing the Mind

There are two tools that I call Hawaiianizing the Mind. One lifts your mind out of the bad neighborhood of stress and transports you to the beach. It's called the PreAttitude Tool. The other transports you to a spa. It's called the Feel It to Heal It Tool.

The PreAttitude Tool

The PreAttitude Tool facilitates a dynamically peaceful attitude in a situation where you might think it wasn't possible. It helps you reframe any difficult situation by infusing it with an attitude of peace. It is conducted prior to engaging the difficult situation, and it offers you the best chance for a successful outcome. In this process, you use the memory of a peaceful and happy time to establish a better attitude toward an upcoming event that makes you anxious, such as a performance review, or in a specific type of situation where you haven't performed as well as you would've liked, such as giving a speech. It may even be a situation in which you have typically disempowered yourself. Through this process you invoke the calm and clarity that will enable you to feel larger than the situation—simply because you are not afraid. By definition, this means you are at peace. And, as you now know, being at peace stimulates higher-brain function, and higher-brain function increases the odds for a more intelligent, creative, and ultimately successful outcome.

I once helped a manager use the PreAttitude Tool to overcome a difficult relationship with a member of her project team. This person had the technical knowledge and skill that were crucial for the team to succeed, but the manager perceived this person as divisive in a way that undermined the collective effort. In several meetings she tried to work out the problem, but those efforts went badly, and they both became defensive and accusatory. It had reached the point where the manager was going to give it one last try, and if the situation didn't go well, she was prepared to fire this person. It was very stressful, and there was a lot at stake on the outcome, but this time she used the PreAttitude Tool to prepare for the meeting. The result was better than she expected.

The PreAttitude Tool helped the manager feel calm, open-minded, and somewhat more positive in the meeting. She was not so focused on the outcome that it interrupted her calm and confidence, especially at the beginning of the meeting when the other person was edgy. She was able to listen to what the other person had to say without any antagonism, which had a calming effect on the other person. The old tension between them dissipated, and for the first time, the two were able to talk constructively about the issue and come up with an approach to improving things.

The Feel It to Heal It Tool

The second tool that Hawaiianizes your mind is the Feel It to Heal It Tool. It's a way of massaging your stressed body with your mind. The purpose of this guided process is to facilitate the relaxation response, which eases the tension that stress has deposited in your body.[1] Stress causes us to tighten muscles. It is part of the freeze response. Becoming more aware of the stress in your body is actually therapeutic and can relieve the tension you're carrying. It also helps you learn the subtle signals of tension in the body and systematically release that tension. Another benefit is that this exercise stimulates alpha brain waves, which, as you'll learn in the next chapter, are a precursor to creative insight.

The process of Feel It to Heal It is simple: you sit comfortably with your eyes closed while you mentally scan your body for tension. The simple act of feeling the tension you're unconsciously holding or ignoring can actually release it. You also penetrate to any emotional state you may be holding, such as some form of grief, fear, or anger. Here, too, simply allowing yourself to feel it can release it. This exercise is particularly helpful in giving your energy a boost in the early or midafternoon when fatigue takes hold, especially on a demanding day.

Your Practice This Week

- Use the PreAttitude Tool in any upcoming difficult situation in which you want to create a positive outcome.
- Perform Feel It to Heal It twice a day, or whenever you notice tension in your body.

And Keep Practicing the Following

- Remember to use the Three Sane Choices Tool if you find yourself feeling powerless in a situation.
- Practice the Thirty-Second Time-Out for Peace Tool three or four times each day.
- Continue using the Getting Clear Tool once every day (twice a day is even better).

- Use the Clear Button Tool to clear a stress-provoking pattern of thinking.
- Continue using the Thought Awareness Tool.
- Continue using the Starting Your Day in Quiet Tool.

Tools

The PreAttitude Tool

- Sit comfortably in your chair with hands free and feet on the ground. Close your eyes and remember a specific place or time when you felt happy and peaceful.
- Make it vivid. See your surroundings. Who are you with, if anyone? Experience how happy and at peace you feel in this setting. Allow yourself to reexperience this good and special moment.
- Next, bring to mind the difficult situation you face. It might be a person or a situation you perceive as difficult or stressful. Imagine that you are in that situation at present. Imagine making the future situation as if it is happening right now. Bring the happy, peaceful feeling you have been visualizing into this situation. See yourself at peace, confident, optimistic, and energetic as you face the situation.
- Imagine that your self-confidence makes you fearless. As a result, you do not give away your sense of personal power. Instead, you feel in charge of your experience. In this fearless state, you are open-minded and not so focused on the outcome that it pulls you away from the peace and confidence you feel. As a result, you feel increasingly larger than the situation simply because you are no longer afraid of it.
- If other people are involved, imagine you are able to communicate what you want to say and listen carefully to what they have to say, with no antagonism toward them.
- Imagine that your sense of calm and clarity remains firm, regardless of what anyone does or doesn't do.

- At the end of the encounter, imagine that you are still at peace, still confident and energetic, whichever way things go.
- Bring your attention to the present moment and, when you are ready, open your eyes.

PreAttitude Tool Guided Process Audio:
A five-minute audio in which Don walks you through the PreAttitude guided process.

http://www.beyondword.com/theendofstress/tag8_Pre -Attitude.mp3

The Feel It to Heal It Tool

- Sit back comfortably in your chair, close your eyes, and allow yourself to feel your body. Notice stress in an area that is particularly uncomfortable, and allow yourself to feel the discomfort, tightness, or tension there. Feel it without imposing any judgment, letting go of the tendency to want to change it. Simply feel it.
- After a few moments, scan your body for tension or discomfort in another place and feel it, again making no judgments about the tension or about yourself. Don't try to change how you feel; simply feel it.
- Keep scanning in this fashion until you have uncovered most of the tension in your body.
- Now see if you can feel your body as a whole. Ask yourself, *How does my whole body feel?*
- Next, imagine for a moment that your body is neutral and that there is an emotional body that can be felt through the physical body. See if you can sense the predominant emotion that emerges. You don't need to name the emotion; simply feel it without imposing any judgment, letting go of the tendency to want to change it.
- Last, allow yourself to gradually relax. Let go of the emotion. Let go of all the tension. Let everything go and relax completely.

- Bring your attention to your breath and follow your breathing for a few breaths. Then open your eyes and look around the room. Take in the colors and shapes of what you see. Be present in a fresh, alert way. Embrace this moment as new and relax into it. Feel the aliveness that is inherent in simple awareness.

Feel It to Heal It Tool Guided Process Audio:
A four-and-a-half-minute audio in which Don walks you through the Feel It To Heal It guided process.

http://www.beyondword.com/theendofstress/tag9_Feel-It -To-Heal-It.mp3

EXPANDING BEYOND STRESS

Keys to Tapping Your Brain's Full Potential

9

The Creative Brain

I n an essay on great men, William James described the brain's creative process as "a seething caldron of ideas, where everything is fizzling and bobbing about in a state of bewildering activity."[1] Science is just beginning to see into the depths of this cauldron and understand how creative insight bubbles up from it. It is becoming clear that some of the old, prevailing notions about creativity are untrue.

Fact #1: Everyone Is Creative

We used to think that people were either genetically gifted with creativity or not, but that's not true. Creativity isn't a function that some have and others don't. Creativity involves a neural network called the anterior superior temporal gyrus, which works in concert with parts of the brain's right hemisphere to generate a creative insight. That insight is then passed to the left hemisphere to be shaped into a practical innovation. These creative processes have been set into everybody's brain, not just a privileged few, but exceptionally creative people have figured out the tricks that activate creative insight. By the end of this chapter, you are going to know the tricks—and, happily, tapping this innate potential is relatively stress free. Simply placing people in a room painted blue can double their creative output. The color blue intimates the sky and the ocean, invoking a more peaceful, happy, and relaxed response. Invoke almost any element of a dynamically peaceful attitude, and you've opened the door to creative insight.

Fact #2: Attention Deficit Feeds Creativity

It was commonly thought that creativity took intense, sustained focus. Again, this is not the case. A number of studies have demonstrated that highly creative people allow a wider range of information into their awareness in contrast to less creative individuals, who tend to focus their attention more narrowly and thereby limit what they experience. A sustained focus is not the best approach when you need a creative solution. A study at the University of Pennsylvania found that so-called smart drugs can keep the brain focused on a problem for eight hours straight, but at the end of the day it isn't likely to deliver any real insights for solving the problem.[2]

Even more telling is a recent study led by Dr. Holly White at the University of Memphis. She found that students diagnosed with attention deficit hyperactivity disorder (ADHD) got significantly higher scores on tests that measured creativity, due in large part to their difficulty with staying focused.[3] White says, "People with ADHD can take an idea and branch it out in lots of different directions. Essentially, ADHD makes them imaginative. By contrast, people without ADHD take a lot of ideas and pull them into a central focus."[4] White also surveyed students who had won prizes at art shows and science fairs. In every field, the students with ADHD had won more awards. Their attention deficit turned out to be a creative blessing. Einstein periodically engaged in what he called thought experiments. He sat quietly in his chair and allowed his mind to wander, sometimes for hours at a time. He reported that it was in this unfocused state that most of his creative insights were born.[5]

Fact #3: Creative Insight Is the Residue of Time Wasted

When I ask a roomful of executives how to sustain competitive edge, most say it's about keeping noses to the grindstone, eyes on the ball, and the company's products on the cutting edge. Certainly, success involves hard work, but the creative insight that leads to cutting-edge innovation requires stepping away from the grind. It's born in the peace and quiet of taking some time off. Yet some of the brightest managers I know shudder at the thought of stimulating innovation by giving upward of a day a week to their employees to use in any way they want. They see it as a colossal waste of time and have difficulty imagining anything productive coming from it. At the same time, every company expects key people to be creative because every company understands that there's no hope of securing a competitive edge without innovation. What most companies don't understand is that when Einstein said "Creativity is the residue of time wasted," he meant that it takes a routine dose of free time for the brain to facilitate the kind of creative insight that leads to breakthroughs in thinking.

One of the first corporations to understand how to facilitate creative insight was 3M, whose long list of innovations is legendary. For decades its employees have been encouraged to use up to 15 percent of their regular work hours to pursue ideas of their own making, even if these ideas are outside 3M's strategic pursuits. It's called the 15-Percent Rule. People are free to do whatever they want with their 15-Percent time, and management trusts that the time will lead to gold, because it has, time and again. The best-known success story of the 15-Percent Rule was scientist Art Fry's creation of Post-its.

He came up with the product on a break while using his 15 percent time to think up ways to bookmark hymns for his church choir. The 15-Percent Rule is so ingrained at 3M that, as one scientist said, "You can feel it right down to your toes."[6] "Daydreaming" is what 3M employees call it. Top management at the company makes it safe to daydream, with few boundaries imposed on how an engineer thinks up a new product.

Other large companies often view 3M's 15-Percent Rule with skepticism. Les Krogh, former senior vice president of research and development at 3M, said, "It was inconceivable that we would permit so much freedom. The 15-Percent philosophy flies in the face of standard management ideas about control."[7] 3M goes as far as to say that innovation is the company's growth engine and that intellectual property is more valuable than "cold cash."[8] But the proof is in the pudding, and in 2012 3M generated $30 billion in sales,[9] filed 3,102 patents, and earned more than $6 a share.[10] Its product line is fifty thousand deep. At last count it has registered nearly twenty-three thousand patents, most of which came from the 15-Percent Rule.[11]

Google is one of the few companies to emulate 3M's approach. Actually, Google upped the ante to 20 percent, and its 20-Percent Rule has provided the same impressive results, giving birth to Gmail and Google Earth.

Fact #4: No Peace, No Joy, No Creative Insight

The tortured artist is a familiar stereotype in our culture, promoting the notion that you have to suffer to create. Well, not according to David Lynch, one of America's great filmmakers, visual artists, and composers.

Lynch says that creativity is not supposed to hurt and that joy is what results in the greatest level of creativity, not pain. Lynch says:

There was a thought for a long time that you had to suffer in order to create, and this is just about opposite of the truth. If you're suffering, even a little bit of suffering cuts into your creativity. In fact, the happier you are, and the more wide awake and rested you are, the better it goes. . . . Then the ideas can flow way better, way smoother and faster, and more of them.[12]

Furthermore, Dr. Mark Beeman of Northwestern University, one of the world's leading researchers on creativity, has found that your mood either blocks or frees creativity. His research has shown that people solve creative problems better when they're in a positive mood.[13] "A positive mood," says Beeman, "might not just relax your scope of interest, but actually broaden it further, allowing you to look at a problem in new ways and come up with a solution."[14] Just watching a YouTube video of a laughing baby was found to increase cognitive flexibility.[15]

American choreographer Martha Graham—whose impact on dance is often compared to that of Picasso on painting, Stravinsky on music, and Frank Lloyd Wright on architecture—said art is built on "an attitude of listening with your whole being,"[16] and "It is your business [as an artist] to keep . . . the channel open."[17]

Neuroscience has identified this channel as the right hemisphere of the brain. We've known about the dichotomy of the right and left brain ever since Roger Sperry, winner of the Nobel Prize in Medicine, defined the split. If you held a human brain in your hands and looked down at it, you would see two separate lobes (or hemispheres) of undulating gray matter positioned side by side. Together they form the cerebral cortex, or higher brain. Although to the naked eye the two lobes are roughly mirror images of each other, they are near polar opposites in the way they function, process information, and behave. The left hemisphere is logical, analytic, quantitative, rational, and literal. It thinks abstractly. It also constructs your individual sense of self as distinct and separate from everything else. The left brain has blessed humanity with science, technology, and most of our social systems, as well as our common sense.

The right hemisphere is conceptual, holistic, intuitive, imaginative, and metaphoric. It thinks in pictures and has blessed humanity with the arts, philosophy, and spirituality, as well as our sense of humor. It also facilitates the profound sense of peace that transcends the separateness that the thinking left brain or "ego" self perceives.

Most of us can recognize the right-brain experience through the change in our mental state whenever we walk out into nature. It's the brain state that naturally arises as you stroll along the ocean shore, close to where the waves are breaking, and breathe in the salt air. Or when you stop in a forest to listen to the rushing sound of the wind and smell the scent of the trees. Or when you traverse a mountain meadow, gliding your hands along the top of the tall grass. You become calmer; your worries, alienation, and grievances fall away; and you begin to feel at one with the world around you. "Nature's peace," John Muir wrote, "will flow into you as sunshine flows into trees. The winds will blow their own freshness into you, and the storms their energy, while cares will drop off like autumn leaves."[18]

The capacity for such experiences is due to that undulating hemisphere of gray matter sitting on the right side of the top of your brain. Turn up its volume with a walk in nature and you're likely to be highly creative for some period afterward. Years ago, a walk in Lassen Volcanic National Park opened that creative channel in me and kept it open for nearly a month. At the time, I had a number of problems that were weighing heavily on me, but as I walked along a stream under a canopy of trees, my heart opened to the beauty surrounding me, and gradually my troubles disappeared. Suddenly, I felt at one with everything. Since my brain surgery, I have had tinnitus, which has produced a never-ending ring in one ear, with the one exception of five beautiful minutes that day by the side of that stream. During this interval, the tinnitus completely vanished. For the first time in fifteen years, I heard with crystal clarity the purity of sound made by Mother Nature. It was like she was singing just for me. I have no idea how my right brain produced that moment—only that it did. I was so filled with the experience that I didn't notice the ringing was gone until it returned. But my heart stayed open. For much of the next month I was as creative as I've ever been. I not only solved most of the problems plaguing me but also produced a book of poetry that eventually made it onto the reading list of a college literature course.

"Each hemisphere," Sperry writes, "seems to have its own separate and private sensations; its own perceptions; its own concepts; and its own impulses to act, with related volitional cognitive and learning experiences."[19] Perhaps the simplest way to characterize the difference between the two brains is to say that the right brain relates to the forest, while the left brain relates to the trees. The two hemispheres communicate with each other across two hundred million nerve fibers called the corpus callosum. When the interplay between the two is harmonious, you access more of your intelligence and are better able to think creatively and turn creative insight into tangible innovation. Some people think of math as strictly a left-brain operation, but a joint study between the US Army and the University of Melbourne found that exceptional ability in math is reached when both the right and left brain work together.[20]

The following table delineates right- and left-brain attributes. Take a moment to reflect on yourself as you navigate through a typical day, then check the brain traits in the table that describe the way you relate to your world and to yourself.

The two hemispheres are like two completely different people who sometimes rub one another the wrong way. One scientist compared the two to the difference between Aristotle (left brain) and Plato (right brain). I think of the two hemispheres as a couple with

RIGHT BRAIN / LEFT BRAIN[21]

	Left Brain	Right Brain
Thinking	Abstract, linear, analytic	Concrete, holistic
Cognitive style	Rational, logical	Intuitive, artistic
Language	Rich vocabulary, good grammar, prosody and syntax, prose	No grammar or syntax, poor vocabulary, metaphorical, poetry
Executive capacity	Introspection, will, initiative, sense of self, focused on the trees	Low sense of self, low initiative, focused on the forest
Specialized functions	Reading, writing, arithmetic, sensory-motor skills, inhibits psychic experience and information	Music, rich dream imagery, good face and gestalt recognition, open to psychic experiences and information
Time experience	Sequentially ordered, measured	Here and now, infinite
Spatial orientation	Relatively poor	Superior, also for shapes, wire figures
Psychoanalytic aspects	Secondary process, ego functions, consciousness	Primary process, dream work, free association

➤ **This worksheet is available for download at theendofstressbook.com/worksheets.**

one partner on the right, the other partner on the left, and the corpus callosum in between providing relationship counseling. Their relationship needs mediation because they're so often at odds. The right brain is the "seething cauldron of ideas" from which creative intelligence emerges, but to the careful and control-driven left brain, right-brain attributes look anything but intelligent.

From a left-brain perspective, the right brain appears a rather wild, emotional, and inarticulate dreamer. Even Roger Sperry didn't have a good thing to say about the right brain in his Nobel Prize acceptance speech. He described the right hemisphere as "relatively retarded" and noted that by contrast to the left hemisphere, it is "not only mute and agraphic but also dyslexic, word-deaf, and apraxic, and lacking generally in higher cognitive function."[22] It's the same sentiment Ralph Kramden barked at Alice in the TV sitcom *The Honeymooners*; Sperry's words are just more erudite. Later, as Sperry's research discovered more about the richness and power of the right brain, his negative view changed completely.

Many of our social systems and institutions are based on the same negative view of right-brain attributes. The scientific revolution placed the left brain high on a pedestal and made our culture left-brain dominant. The industrial and information revolutions that followed fortified its dominance. As a result, the creative, intuitive, emotional, artistic right brain is often subjugated. This explains why men have believed women are inferior, the status quo distrusts the avant-garde, and our schools suffer from what the German educational reformer Wilhelm Reese called "the hypertrophy of the intellect and the atrophy of the imagination and heart."[23]

Our left-brain culture has become increasingly dissociated from that inner realm from which creativity and beauty emanate. You can see it in our art and architecture. You can hear it in our music and read it in our literature. The ugliness of the modern world surrounds us. When I take the train out of Grand Central Station north toward West Point or the BART from Berkeley into San Francisco, I am struck by the long stretches of ugliness that meet the eye. Even when the landscape breaks free from the urban blight that the left brain engineered, the open space is scarred like a pockmarked face.

The superior intellect, verbal skill, and drive of the left hemisphere, when it dominates, can overpower right-brain activity, shutting it out. It comes at great cost. Lose right-brain function and you lose the intuitive feel that knows what to do when your intellect doesn't. Shut out the right brain and you lose that magical capacity to free-associate your way through a haystack of unrelated facts, images, and memories to find the needle. Without the right brain, the left brain fills with dots it can't connect. You won't be adept at reading people's faces or deciphering their intentions. Your own voice will lack intonation, and you'll be inept at expressing emotion. And if that weren't bad enough, without the right brain, figurative language will be lost on you. Only the literal meanings of words will make sense to you. As a result, you won't get jokes, metaphors, irony, sarcasm, jargon, or figures of speech. These subtleties of language will sail right over your left brain's head. You won't get the point of a story, the meaning in a poem, or the aesthetic of a painting, and you won't be aroused by music. You'll possess none of the playfulness or inhibition that turns into artistry. And, perhaps most tragic of all, you'll be incapable of reaching the depth of inner peace that opens to the experience of oneness.

That's a lot to give up for just intellect. It's why in an interview Ray Bradbury asserted that "thinking is the enemy of creativity." His advice was, "Don't think. . . . You solve problems not by thinking directly of them but allowing them to ferment in their own time."[24]

Another way of saying this is leave creativity to the right brain. Einstein felt much the same way. He said that words, which are the domain of the left brain, did not seem to play any role in his mechanism of creative thought. Rather, he said, he saw his ideas in pictures, which arise from the right brain. It seemed to Einstein that the essential feature of "productive thought" first came in the form of signs and more or less clear images that he played with first before turning them into the language that could communicate the idea to others.[25]

John Kounios of Drexel University, one of the world's leading researchers on the brain and creativity, defines creative insight as the sudden awareness of the solution to a problem, with little or no understanding of how it happened.[26] Insight essentially dawns on us. When most of us turn our attention to solving a tricky problem that requires creative insight, the left hemisphere initially takes charge. It makes an intense mental search in a linear, intellectual, task-oriented manner, but as it turns out, the left brain's approach does not generate the necessary insight that solves a mind-twisting problem.

Researchers discovered this by using a word puzzle to test the basic mechanisms at work during creative insight. The puzzle is called the Remote Associates Test (if you're interested in taking this test, you will find a copy of it at the end of this chapter). Subjects are given three different words and asked to find a single word that works with each in a compound word phrase. For example, the solution to the puzzle *beef*, *glass*, and *hog* is ground, as in ground beef, ground glass, and groundhog. The problem the left brain has with the puzzle is that it doesn't possess the right brain's ability to see the relationship between the seemingly remote and unrelated fragments that connect up to form a whole, meaning the single word that solves a given problem on the Remote Associates Test. The left brain isn't adept at associating one fragment with another. It gets stuck in the trees, as opposed to the right brain, which can see the forest through the trees.

Dr. Mark Beeman's research found that nearly all the solutions to the Remote Associates Test that the left brain came up with were wrong. He found that when you use intellect to solve a problem that requires creative insight, you usually end up stumped. Your left brain draws blanks, and you eventually give up the effort. Ironically, when you stop trying to get the answer, it often arrives like sunlight breaking through the clouds. In the moment of impasse, the right brain picks up the problem the left brain has dropped. Activity diverges from the left to the right brain to explore the problem in a spontaneous, free-flowing, and nonlinear manner.[27]

To put it in Zen terms, the left brain stops trying to figure it out, which allows the right brain the chance to feel its way to the answer. There is a burst of alpha wave activity from the right brain, signaling some form of turning inward. Alpha wave activity increases when the brain takes a break from goal-directed tasks, but it doesn't mean your mind is a void.[28] It's actually working hard. One-third of a second before the solution pops into your head, there is a burst of gamma wave activity on the right side of the brain. Gamma waves spike when higher-brain processes are engaged. The gamma wave rhythm gathers and binds together perceptions, thoughts, associations, and memories to form a novel idea, like the answer to a tricky problem. When the flash of gamma waves happens, your slouched posture of defeat suddenly straightens up, your eyes sparkle, and you shout "Aha!" The neural integration that leads to the sudden insight emerges from a moment of simply standing still to see what rises up from the quiet depths of the right brain.

Stop and Stand Still

Generating creative insight is a matter of moving the left brain out of the way for a short time. This is accomplished by stopping and becoming still within in order to see what creative insight rises up from the right brain. There is a wonderful quote about stopping and standing still that comes from Lee Ufan, one of the world's great present-day artists. Ufan is addressing all of us when he says, "Agitated, busy people. Stop and stand still for just a moment. Look at the blue sky. Close your eyes and take a deep breath. If you will just do this, you will change, and the world will come to life."[29] There are several simple but proven tools for stopping and standing still in order to open the channel for creative insight.

Stop and Stand Still Tool #1:
Invite moments of creative insight by taking breaks and going on walks in a green setting.
This is one of the most important things you can do during the day to stimulate creative insight. Some of the world's greatest break-

throughs happened when the left brain took a break and unwittingly made room for the right brain to work its magic. One of the most famous accounts is of James Watt, the Scottish inventor, whose improvements to the steam engine were fundamental to launching the Industrial Revolution. Every attempt Watt made to perfect the steam engine had failed, until one day, on reaching yet another impasse, he gave up. Then he went for a walk to get away from it all. As he relaxed, suddenly he experienced a profound, out-of-the-blue moment of insight that perfected the steam engine. He said, "I had not walked farther than the Golf-house . . . when the whole thing was arranged in my mind."[30]

Breaks create the brain state in which the dots connect themselves. Breaks also improve memory and support what is called "memory consolidation," which is essential to envisioning something novel or learning something new. Nathan Kleitman, considered the father of sleep research, discovered what is called the basic rest-activity cycle (BRAC).[31] This cycle repeats itself about every ninety minutes. During the first half of the BRAC, brain waves oscillate at a fast rate. You feel wide awake and are able to focus your attention. During the last half, your brain waves start to slow down until, in the last twenty minutes of BRAC, you begin to feel day-dreamy and somewhat tired.[32]

During the fast–brain wave phase, each brain cell uses sodium and potassium ions to generate electrical signals. But the fast brain waves burn through these ions, which means your brain requires a period of rest to restore the sodium-potassium balance. The restoration process can require up to twenty minutes of rest, after which your brain rebounds with the fuel to run fast brain waves. Kleitman found that human beings perform best in a permanent cycle of ninety minutes of activity followed by a period of rest. It's how we human beings actually get more done.

Related research has found that BRAC's ninety-minute cycle is the best way to achieve mastery. This discovery was made by Anders

Ericsson, who studied people who had become expert performers. In particular, Erickson's research team focused on young violinists who were considered to be the best of the best. He found these violinists universally limited the rigors of practice to ninety-minute sessions, systematically distributed over the day, followed by a leisurely break, and sometimes even an afternoon nap.[33]

Most people can't imagine stepping away from work every ninety minutes. Part of this reaction is guilt. Breaks can make people feel like truants. They can also induce the anxiety that thinks a break will cause us to fall behind. For some, the good sense of taking a break is overwhelmed by the obsessive compulsion that keeps our nose to the grindstone. We need to change that mind-set to reflect the science. Taking a break means you're becoming more productive, with greater creative insight and mastery, not less.

This doesn't mean you have to take a break when you're on a roll. The important thing is to monitor your mental energy before it hits bottom. What depletes mental energy most is pushing yourself to keep going when you sense that the ions fueling your effort are nearly spent.

If you can't imagine taking a break every ninety minutes, then start by taking a break midmorning and another midafternoon. If possible, connect with nature, either by looking out a window or by going outside. As you take your break, be sure to keep a porthole open in your mind to let in any creative insight. I guarantee that the creative insight and improved brain function you will experience will motivate you to add more breaks to your day.

In addition, take a twenty- to thirty-minute walk a couple of times a week in a green setting. Research has found that moderate walking three times per week for a year increased brain connectivity and brain function.[34] Walking feeds the brain with ample amounts of oxygen and glucose that the large muscles devour during aerobic exercise. Glucose and oxygen are the fuel on which the brain runs.

Furthermore, a study at the University of Essex found that just a small dose of nature every day will benefit people's mood, self-esteem, and mental health. The conclusion was drawn from ten studies conducted in the United Kingdom, working with more than twelve hundred subjects from a wide demographic range. It revealed that activity in nature—what researchers dubbed "green exercise"—resulted in significant health benefits.[35] Green exercise is walking in a park, gardening, cycling, fishing, boating, horseback riding, and farming.

One of the studies found that *green* really matters. This study took twenty people with depression and compared the benefits of a thirty-minute walk in a country park with a walk in an indoor shopping mall. After the country walk, 71 percent reported decreased levels of depression and said they felt less tense, while 90 percent reported increased self-esteem. In contrast, only 45 percent experienced a decrease in depression after the shopping center walk. Green exercise is now considered a clinically valid treatment option for people experiencing mental distress.

Finally, take a real lunch break away from your desk. A study from Germany found that having lunch at a restaurant with colleagues or friends is more relaxing than a meal eaten alone at your desk.[36] People who eat at their desk usually work all hour, while people who lunch with friends are more likely to let go of work. As a result, they are more refreshed and more creative when they return to the office.

Stop and Stand Still Tool #2:
Make the space to let your imagination wander.

A study by Benjamin Baird and Jonathan Schooler at the University of California at Santa Barbara suggests that simple tasks that allow the mind to wander may facilitate creative problem solving. In the study, subjects worked on solving problems that required creativity. After a testing session, Baird divided subjects into three groups and gave them a so-called rest period. However, the research team kept one of the groups busy with a demanding task that engaged their brains. The second group was assigned an easy, somewhat mindless task that predictably led to mind-wandering. The third group was given no task at all. After the break, they all went back to work on the creative problem-solving exercise. When the results were tabulated, it was the mind-wanderers who solved more problems.[37] This helps explain why the 15-Percent Rule at 3M works, and why 3M employees call it daydreaming.

So don't be afraid to let your mind wander every now and then. Just be sure to maintain enough awareness to catch a creative thought swimming to shore from the ocean of a right-brain daydream.

Stop and Stand Still Tool #3:
If the solution to a problem eludes you, sleep on it.

In the morning, check in with your right brain to see if it has any insight to offer. You can build this check-in process into the Starting the Day in Quiet Tool, which you should already be doing (or, if you haven't begun it yet, here's a second chance to start). Researchers have found that insights often happen just before you go to sleep or early in the morning, shortly after waking up.[38] The brain's right hemisphere is more active than normal at these times. The relaxed, dreamy, and seemingly unorthodox state of your brain makes you open to all sorts of out-of-the box ideas.

Unfortunately, most people don't take advantage of this window into the brain's cauldron of creativity. Morning for most people is rushed, and as a result they miss a possible insight. One morning, Elias Howe, the inventor of the sewing machine, didn't rush on waking. Instead, he sat up in bed and mused over a dream his right brain had generated the night before. He dreamed that he was running for his life from a band of cannibals, who were gaining on him. When he turned to see how close the cannibals had come, he noticed that the blades of their spears had holes near the blade's tip. As he pondered the dream that morning, he had a sudden flash of insight. The holes in the spears resembled the eye of the needle he used in his failed sewing machine, with one difference: the eye on his machine was in the middle of the needle's shaft, not at the tip. He ran to his lab and moved the eye to the tip of the needle to match his dream, and lo and behold, the sewing machine was invented.

The moral of the story is to wake up a little earlier, ahead of the rush. Take a few moments and open to your right brain. See if it has anything to offer. You can easily add this to the beginning of the Starting the Day in Quiet exercise you learned in chapter 2. Upon waking, sit up in bed and take a moment to see whether the right brain has anything to offer, especially if you have a difficult problem you haven't been able to solve. After a few moments of listening with quiet receptivity, go to that part of the house where you have been starting your day in quiet and do the usual exercise, which is to invoke a positive, peaceful attitude to frame a great day.

Stop and Stand Still Tool #4:
Occasionally, take time to increase your
alpha wave activity by counting your blessings.

Recent research has found that people who are more grateful have higher levels of happiness and well-being.[39] As I previously said, people who score high on a standard measure of happiness are more creative than people who are feeling stressed. Unhappiness drops your chances of creative insight to slightly below random chance,[40] meaning that if you have a creative thought, it was an accident. So give yourself a creative leg up by counting your blessings.

Sonja Lyubomirsky, an experimental psychologist at the University of California at Riverside, found that people who once a week wrote down things they were grateful for were happier than those who did it three times a week. "When people do anything too often," Dr. Lyubomirsky speculates, "it loses the freshness and meaning."[41] So once a week, recall three things that happened during the previous week for which you are grateful. Then acknowledge three things in your life for which you feel blessed.

Kick-Starting the Right Brain

In addition to everything I've outlined so far, you can shift your right brain into creative high gear by doing some things that may seem rather silly—but they work.

Laughing: If you feel your creative power is ebbing, increase your feeling of happiness by doing something that makes you laugh. You can accomplish this by going to YouTube to search for the videos of babies laughing. Believe me: they'll have you laughing out loud. The videos are not only funny, they're heartwarming. They'll make you'll feel brighter and happier, which will give your creative intelligence an immediate boost. You can get the same lift from watching an episode of your favorite sitcom or listening to your favorite comedian.

Painting the walls blue: As I already mentioned, painting your office, study, or studio a soft shade of blue has been proven to stimulate the right brain to increase creative insight.

Squeezing a ball: Believe it or not, squeezing a ball in your left hand has also been shown to activate the right brain (your right brain controls your left side, and vice versa). In one study, two groups of participants took the Remote Associates Test after squeezing a ball. One group squeezed the ball with their left hand; the other group squeezed with their right hand. The hypothesis was that left-hand contractions caused right-brain activation, leading to better scores on the Remote Associates Test.[42] It worked, improving scores by as much as 50 percent. A study by Ruth Propper corroborated these findings.[43] So give it try. Purchase a two-inch solid rubber ball, the kind typically used as a fetch toy for dogs. Hold the ball in your left hand and squeeze it hard for two sets of forty-five seconds each. Be sure to take a fifteen-second break between sets. Then turn your attention back to the problem or project at hand that requires a boost in creativity.

Taking a trip: Taking an occasional weekend sojourn to someplace new and interesting can stimulate your right brain. Traveling in a foreign country can turn up your creative energy even more, and living for an extended period in a foreign country can have an even bigger effect. All the new and exciting experiences that traveling generates spike creative insight and output. We all know about Ernest Hemingway, F. Scott Fitzgerald, Gertrude Stein, and Picasso leaving their native lands to live as expatriates in Paris, and it turns out that these artists knew what they were doing. Five different studies have explored the link between living abroad and creative genius and found it to be consistent across a number of creativity measures.[44]

Taking a Walk: Walking is a robust solution to increasing creativity when your creative well has run dry. Researchers at Stanford University studied creative divergent thinking while walking versus sitting in more than 170 people. They found that a person's creative output increased by an average of 60 percent when walking.[45] Walking opens up the free flow of ideas, and creative thinking continues even after you're back at your desk. Beethoven wrote symphonies in his head while on long walks, and Steve Jobs preferred to conduct creative meetings on walks.

Your Practice This Week

MY COMMITMENT		
Fill out the form below and begin practicing all three items.		
I commit to waking up each morning	_____ minutes earlier	to start the day on a positive note.
I commit to counting my blessings once a week, every week	on this day: _____	Beginning: / /
Each day I will take a break at:	_____ in the morning	_____ in the afternoon

➤ **This worksheet is available for download at theendofstressbook.com/worksheets.**

And Keep Practicing the Following

- Use the Three Sane Choices Tool if you are feeling powerless in a situation and Feel It to Heal It if tension is mounting in your body.
- Practice the Thirty-Second Time-Out for Peace a few times daily.
- Continue using the Getting Clear Tool once daily (twice is better).
- Use the Clear Button Tool to clear a stress-provoking thinking pattern.
- Continue using the Thought Awareness Tool.
- Continue starting your day in quiet. Wake up a bit earlier to explore any insights the right brain brewed up while you were asleep.

Tools

The Stop and Stand Still

The Stop and Stand Still Tool invites a moment of creative insight.

- Take breaks every couple of hours. Go for walks in a green setting.
- Make the space to let your imagination wander.
- If the solution to a problem eludes you, sleep on it. When you wake up, sit back and see if you've received an answer.
- Once a week, count your blessings.

Take the Remote Associates Test

You are given three different words (the triad). The task is to find a single word that can form a compound word or phrase that works with all three words. For example, consider the triad age, mile, and sand. The solution is stone (stone age, milestone, sandstone).

REMOTE ASSOCIATES TEST[46]*	
TRIAD	**SOLUTION**
Notch, flight, spin	
Speak, money, street	
Sandwich, golf, foot	
Cotton, bathtub, tonic	
Sore, shoulder, sweat	
Ink, herring, neck	

*Answers: 1. Top. 2. Easy. 3. Club. 4. Gin. 5. Cold. 6. Red.

➤ **This worksheet is available for download at theendofstressbook.com/worksheets.**

10

Vacations Heal the Brain Damage from Last Year's Stress

Along with taking breaks every day, you need to take a vacation. A joint study of the University of Minho in Portugal and the Laboratory for Integrative Neuroscience at the National Institutes of Health (NIH) suggests that a vacation is critical to restoring higher-brain function that shows signs of failing because of prolonged exposure to stress.[1] In this study, rats were divided into two groups: one that would be chronically stressed and one that wouldn't. Prior to beginning the study, both groups were trained to press a lever to receive food rewards, and once they were proficient at it, researchers changed the situation by feeding the animals by hand, sparing them the effort of pressing the lever. This meant both groups were getting the food essentially for free.

Then the study subjected one group of rats to a constant condition of stress over twenty-one days in a random, unpredictable manner. The rats didn't know when the next assault was coming, making conditions even more stressful. Researchers shocked the rats with moderate jolts of electricity, submerged them in water, and exposed them to the bullying of alpha male rats. As a result of their stressful life, the rats stopped behaving intelligently. Their brain completely forgot about the hand-delivered food and resorted to pressing the lever over and over again. They'd lost access to the knowledge of a better approach. The researchers also found that the change in behavior was reflected in brain structure. On the one hand, the buildup of stress hormones shrank and atrophied higher-order networks associated with executive decision making and goal-directed behaviors. On the other hand, it fortified more primitive networks linked to habit formation. Habits formed from stress reactions are usually bad habits. The result was a brain caught in an endlessly looping algorithm of inefficient and unproductive behaviors that the brain was unable to detect and correct.

"Behaviors become habitual faster in stressed animals," stated the head of the study, Dr. Nuno Sousa. "Worse, the stressed animals can't shift back to goal-directed behaviors when that would be the better approach."[2] You lose that capacity when you are chronically stressed. Your beleaguered brain locks you into doing the same unproductive things again and again. You eventually dig yourself into a rut and can't find your way out.

But there is good news in this otherwise bleak picture. The researchers found that the problem is reversible. Just four weeks of vacation from their stress-provoking environment were enough for neuroplasticity to heal the rats' brains. Higher-brain networks resprouted, blossoming with the intelligence to function successfully, and the overgrown networks habituating dysfunction were pruned back. The brain is quite resilient if given the chance to rebound. It can reverse the damage stress has caused and build new structures to increase your capacity to succeed at life.

But for positive neuroplasticity to work its magic, you have to give the brain time to heal, which means a vacation. The brain needs you to step away for a while from the stress of the previous year. Unfortunately, this is not what a lot of people are doing. More than a third of employees in the United States aren't planning to take their full vacation. Of those who do take vacations, only 14 percent go away for two weeks or more at any one time.[3] Of those who do go away, 82 percent will check in with the office at least once a day, 40 percent will check multiple times each day, and 37 percent will come fully equipped with smartphones, laptops, and tablets.[4]

An article in *The New York Times* reported the account of a Manhattan publicist taking her first official vacation in four years. "As soon as her plane landed," the article reported, "she checked her phone for work messages. Upon arriving at her hotel, the first thing she did was locate the business center."[5] Then she spent much of the first two days in her room sulking over weather conditions. She didn't stop checking her email and phone messages for the rest of her time on the trip. This describes the new normal for vacations.

Recently I took at a vacation on the Monterey Peninsula. I was standing on the dunes just above the beach, looking out over the magnificent scenery, and I was surprised to see a number of adult vacationers looking down at their smartphones, not at the sea and sky, while around them, kids were pecking away at handheld devices instead of building sand castles.

This is not giving the brain the break it requires to recover from how hard it was pushed last year. We should think of vacation as a neurological intensive care unit, where our condition requires that we be sequestered from the stress and strain of the outside world.

It takes a kind of mental discipline to let go of the office and open our minds to the renewal that a mix of leisure and adventure can generate. We may be afraid that our workload will grow exponentially while we're away, or that some ambitious understudy will dazzle the boss in our absence and steal our job. It takes courage to let go of those fears and wake up to the biological evidence encouraging us to leave the job behind for a few weeks. If you do, the evidence says you'll return to work with a brand new brain generating the cerebral power to produce your best year ever.

A Vacation Guide for Healing Your Brain

Before you leave, make the goal of your vacation to succeed at extending love, feeling at peace, and experiencing joy. All three are good medicine for the brain. Be certain to make a plan with an assistant or trusted colleague at work for contacting you in the case of something urgent. Then set up your email account with an autoresponder and create email and voice messages that refer people to your office contact for urgent issues.

Once you arrive at your destination, commit to using your smartphone for local calls only, not routine calls to the office. Use your tablet for reading books and playing solitaire, not for work. If you have to use a work device, be disciplined about it. It should only be for a pressing, unavoidable issue. Let nonurgent business messages go to voice mail, and don't let yourself get sucked into emails by reading them first thing in the morning.

Start each day in quiet. Allow your heart and mind to open wide to the freshness and freedom a vacation engenders. Make it a practice to quiet any obsession you might have with electronic devices. Look up from the device and take in the world around you. Remind yourself that your smartphone isn't the place where your vacation is happening.

Be present, right here, right now. Let go of the past and future whenever it raises its stress-provoking head. Let go of worries and judgments. Commit to tuning in to the loved ones who are with you. Take the opportunity to discover them all over again. Lean into appreciating them.

What to Do if You Can't Afford a Vacation?

I understand that money, time, family constraints, and business pressures can thwart a vacation. Even so, your brain needs the recovery time, so think creatively about how to get some rest and relaxation. It's too important, especially if you've had a stressful year. Where there is a will, there is a way. Below are three suggestions, but don't limit yourself to these. Whatever you choose to do in taking care of your brain, the key is making the effort to stay off the work calls, turn off emails, and follow the Vacation Guide for Healing Your Brain that I just outlined.

1. **A four- to five-day getaway:** As I mentioned in the creative brain section, getting away for a few days can kick-start creativity. Extending your weekend by two or three days will give you the recovery time to bring your stress level down, which will help your brain.
2. **Staycations:** A staycation is the new buzzword for something people have been doing for hundreds of years: taking their vacations at home. A staycation can give the brain the time it needs to repair, but you might have to be more diligent about keeping the office at bay. If you have children and your home has a backyard, you can set up a campsite, tent and all, and spend a night or two camping out and stargazing with the kids.
3. **House swapping:** You can give yourself a vacation that is a cut above a staycation by virtue of landing in a new environment. This involves swapping your home with someone you trust who also needs an alternative plan for a vacation.

Your Practice This Week

This week make a plan for your vacation, even if it's still months away. Plan when you want to take the time off. Think of where you want to go, or decide on an alternative plan if there is a money or other issue to consider. Begin to make the arrangements that will make your vacation happen. Your brain will thank you.

Keep Practicing the Following

- Remember to use the Three Sane Choices Tool if you find yourself feeling powerless in a situation and Feel It to Heal It if you find tension mounting in your body.
- Practice the Thirty-Second Time-Out for Peace Tool a few times each day.
- Continue using the Getting Clear Tool once every day (twice a day is even better).
- Use the Clear Button Tool to clear a stress-provoking pattern of thinking.
- Continue using the Thought Awareness Tool.
- Continue using the Start Your Day in Quiet Tool, waking up a little earlier to explore any insights the right brain brewed up while you were asleep.
- Put the Stop and Stand Still Tool to use: Take breaks. Go for walks in a green setting. If you have a difficult problem, sleep on it and in the morning see whether there is an answer to it that your brain dreamed up. Once a week, count your blessings.

11

The Whole of You That Transcends the Fragments

A friend of mine went through a difficult period over several months when her company was having cash flow problems. She repeatedly had to rob Peter to pay Paul, which bothered her sense of integrity and stressed her. One day, when the anxiety about her problem happened to be especially high, she went to the ATM to draw some pocket cash. As she slipped her card into the slot, she suddenly experienced a flash of extreme stress and fear. For a moment, she fantasized about the machine opening and an FBI agent stepping out to arrest her for impersonating an honest human being. Of course, this was absurd, and my friend laughed at it, albeit nervously.

More than likely, this stress reaction was caused by shame. Shame can make your heart pound and leave you feeling shaky and vulnerable. The fantasy of being arrested is another example of how insanely the lower brain makes us think when we're chronically stressed, just as it did with the salesman in the What Am I Afraid Of? exercise. The fear of being seen as having failed, whether we've actually failed or not, can excite the fear of being banished.

Shame is the key emotional response we feel when we are threatened by some kind of social evaluation or social rejection. Sigmund

Freud defined shame as the kind of social anxiety that leads peo-ple to being controlled by what others think and say about them.[1] The research of Brené Brown of the University of Houston found that "shame is all about fear . . . the fear of disconnection," which she describes as "the fear of being perceived as flawed and unwor-thy of acceptance or belonging."[2] As you now know, fear invariably means stress.

Shame produces the insidious, haunting thought that says there's something fraudulent or wrong about us, something that must be kept hidden, for if others were to discover it, they would run us out of town. Shame is built on layers of self-contempt and unworthi-ness that were programmed into our self-view during our formative years, when parents harped on our faults, friends and siblings ridi-culed us, and coaches and teachers ignored or criticized our talents and efforts. It is the root of dysfunction in families and plays a role in social phobias, eating disorders, domestic violence, schoolyard bullies, and substance abuse.[3] It develops from a repetitive, negative pattern of self-effacement that etches into the brain to produce the self-perpetuating thought *I'm not good enough*. Eventually, it dark-ens into the self-defeating belief *I'm not good enough because there is something wrong with me*. The emotional weight of this is too heavy for our minds to carry, so we repress it to a dark corner of the mind, where it festers. The picture that shame paints represents a life that is the polar opposite of flourishing. It thwarts us from functioning fully, which Carl Rogers, the father of humanistic psychology, described as a person "moving in the direction of wholeness, integration, a unified life . . . toward fulfillment [and] actualization."[4]

We've all experienced social anxiety while being evaluated. In my case, I get evaluated often, at the end of every corporate seminar I conduct. Evaluation time used to be stressful for me. If forty-eight people rated the seminar good to outstanding and two rated it aver-age or poor, my brain would fixate on the two unhappy scores. The lower scores made me feel insecure, as if I hadn't been good enough. It was ridiculous. After one training, my business partner challenged me to read the positive evaluations and let them affect me. I actually had a hard time taking in the good comments. It was a wake-up call for me to get to the bottom of these shame-based stress reactions.

Make no mistake, shame is stressful. The fear of being criticized, judged, rejected, or devalued in any way is extremely stressful. Its effect on our body and ultimately our health and well-being can be even more pernicious than work stress. "People think that all stresses have the same effect on the body," writes Dr. Margaret Kemeny of the University of California at San Francisco, "but stress caused by how others view you is extremely powerful, as much or more so than those caused from . . . working too hard."[5] Her study, which appeared in the *Journal of Personality,* found that "acute threats to our social self increase stress hormones and proinflammatory cytokine activity occurring in concert with shame."[6] "Acute threats" refers to the pain of being criticized or rejected. The increase in stress hormones and proinflammatory cytokine activity means that shame-related stress reactions can dampen higher-brain function and can eventually make you seriously ill.

Shame is social anxiety, and anxiety triggers stress reactions. The stress response system is wired to react to threats, especially threats to our social self. Back when our species lived out in the wilds, a threat to our social position could mean banishment from the tribe, and that meant certain death. Thus, to the amygdala, the brain's fear center, a social threat is a serious survival issue and reason to activate the stress response system. But we're not in the wilds anymore, and the good news in all this bad news about shame is that we can rewire our brains to respond differently. "By developing the ability to focus our attention on our internal world," states neuropsychiatrist Daniel Siegel, "we are picking up a 'scalpel' we can use to re-sculpt our neural pathways, stimulating the growth of areas of the brain that are crucial to mental health."[7] In other words, neuroplasticity can rewire our brain to alleviate shame. In this chapter, we are going to approach rewiring the brain to open the door wide to the whole of you, instead of all the fragmentation shame causes.

Building Awareness

Over the years, researchers have explored the stressful waters of shame, and what they've found can help us become more aware of what drives shame so we can change it. Carol Dweck, one of the world's leading researchers in emotional development, found that shame's encoding process starts early in life. She conducted a study of third-graders to try to explain why kids fail in school. She found that boys who failed at an assignment were routinely told "You weren't paying attention" or "You didn't make the effort."

Girls were routinely told "You're not very good at arithmetic" or "You're sloppy and don't check your work." Dweck conducted an experiment with students in which she gave them an unsolvable word puzzle. When she asked the children why they hadn't solved the puzzle, the boys acted as if they didn't care. Some got angry and called the puzzle stupid. The girls became self-effacing, offering some version of "I'm not very bright."[8]

Since Dweck's experiment, studies on shame have found that this same pattern continues into adulthood. Shame-based stress in men tends to turn shame into anger, causing a "shame-anger feed-back loop."[9] Men get caught in a vicious cycle of feeling ashamed at being angry, and being angry at feeling ashamed. Sometimes the overstimulated amygdala erupts in violence. According to psychiatrist Donald Nathanson, every incident of domestic violence can be traced back to shame.[10]

On the other hand, shame-based stress in women follows a "shame-shame feedback loop."[11] Women essentially feel ashamed of feeling ashamed, which makes them more ashamed, exciting stress reactions. Eventually, the circuitous process turns into depression.

In both men and women, shame represents a psychoneurological pattern that activates pernicious stress reactions and holds the better angels of human nature hostage. This is the first piece in the pattern to bring into awareness. It means catching the first signs of shame and observing how the vicious pattern unfolds, shame erupting in anger for men and shame multiplying shame in women. The Thought Awareness Tool can be helpful, first in detecting a state of shame and next in dispelling the beliefs that cause it to escalate. Awareness is key. In chapter 3, I laid out how simple awareness can open the door to rewire what's been hardwired into the brain. The same applies to a brain wired for shame.

The Shame Exercise

So let's get up close and personal with shame by doing a simple exercise that increases awareness. Imagine that you have had a great day. You brought some project to a successful conclusion, and you are elated. You can't wait to share your success at a meeting that's about to take place. Make that feeling of excitement as vivid as you can. Now see yourself at that meeting with people sitting around the table. You enthusiastically share the day's success, expecting your colleagues to join in your revelry and congratulate you. But they don't. When you've finished telling them about your success, no one responds other than to nod their head, and then someone summarily changes the subject. There is no joining in your elation. Instead, your tale of success is met with disinterest.

How would this make you feel? How would it color your success? How would this color the way you feel about yourself?

If this situation were to actually happen to you, it's likely it would cause a shame reaction. Your elation would instantly evaporate.

Initially, you'd feel distressed, then inhibited, and ultimately embarrassed about making a point of your success. You'd want to disappear into the woodwork. Afterward, you might feel hurt and angry, and eventually depressed, reinforcing your sense of unworthiness. Shame takes other people's indifference or insensitivity to heart. It interprets it to mean *There is something wrong with me*. In this case, your shame would be produced by this rapid transition from a happy state to a painful state, which involves a collision of the sympathetic and parasympathetic nervous systems.[12]

The feelings of elation over succeeding at the project, along with the excitement of wanting to share it, arouse the sympathetic nervous system. This system is the brain's accelerator pedal, revving up the motor. When you're elated, it generates an internal YES to life.

The parasympathetic nervous system throws on the brakes. It's the effect of others who weren't interested in your success. This affront generates a sudden stop that abruptly ends your elation. This is an external NO extinguishing your internal YES. I often refer to this collision of YES and NO as the Sympathetic-Parasympathetic Crash.

I Made a Mistake Exercise

Let's do another exercise to generate awareness around an experience of shame when we make a mistake. Imagine that you've created a budget projection for the next six months of a program that projects a surplus. You've sent a summary to your boss stating that cuts to the program are unnecessary because of the surplus. The next day you discover that some of the calculations in your projection are wrong and, once corrected, show a troubling deficit. You sit there alone, aware that it's your mistake and that you have to tell the boss. What do you imagine you would be saying to yourself? At times I found myself in this very position when I managed large organizations, and the harsh words I called myself are not fit for print.

This shame-filled, red-pencil mind-set berates us with could have, should have, would haves that we direct at ourselves and project onto other people. We chronically should all over ourselves, as the pun goes. We also should on other people, and they should on us. This can't help but trigger a fight, flight, or freeze reaction in a brain wired for shame.

The "Ideal Self"

Carl Rogers found that shame manufactures what he called the "ideal self."[13] By ideal, Rogers is not suggesting a better self, but rather a sense of self that is not real, something inauthentic. It's a breeding ground for shame. It's the image of the ideal person we think we should be who is always out of reach—the standard we can never meet. It represents the gap between the authentic self and the ideal self, between the "I am" and the "I should be." The gap produces incongruity in our sense of self that, in turn, produces a feeling of inadequacy that has us asking, *Who am I?* We end up lost, and there is nothing more stressful than being lost.

Albert Ellis, the founder of cognitive behavioral therapy, found that the essence of what we call neurosis is at the bottom of three shame-based sentences that people tell themselves.

1. The first sentence is *I made a mistake; I made an error, and I got it wrong*. This may invoke feelings of guilt or frustration, but if we were to stop here, the crisis would only represent an error to correct or a lesson to learn, extending the opportunity to grow or advance.

2. The second sentence is *This mistake I made . . . This event that turned out badly . . . This thing I got wrong . . . This way I behaved . . . it means that there's something wrong with me*. This is guilt or frustration becoming shame. It has us saying to ourselves *I'm not*

good enough; I'm not smart enough; I'm not worthy enough; I'm not loveable enough, all of which calcify into the belief that *I'm no good and deserve whatever punishment is coming*. Albert Ellis defines this reaction as the moralistic condemnation of yourself as an individual. "It is a complete confusion," Ellis states, "between the individual and his or her act or behavior. And it is this sentence . . . that I'm no good—that does the damage."[14]

3. The third sentence is *I am going to do wrong again, and make even bigger mistakes*. In other words, we lose confidence in ourselves.[15]

It reaches the point where we're afraid to make a mistake, more because of the emotional punishment we know we will inflict on ourselves than for anything the world might do to us.

Eventually, a shame-based mind represses its mistakes to avoid feeling bad, preventing the possibility of learning from a mistake, which only increases the likelihood of repeating the blunder. Our mistakes can't teach us anything; they can't grow into knowledge. The problem with repression is that it isn't selective. We can't numb ourselves to difficult feelings, such as shame, without numbing ourselves to great feelings, like joy, passion, and peace. Repression dulls the brain's emotional system, which eventually bottoms out as depression.

It gets even worse. It means we also can't see what's right about us, and we end up holding to a narrow view of our strengths, talents, and contributions. Herbert Otto's groundbreaking research on human potential found that most people can list only five or six good points about themselves, but can fill one to two pages with what they perceive as their faults.[16] When the Gallup organization asked American workers to identify their strengths, one-third could not name any.[17]

Until this changes, there can be no joy in our work, no pride in our achievements, and no peace in our hearts. There can be no real understanding of who we are and can become. A life defined by shame is predictably stressful and unfulfilling. It is a life unable to realize its full potential.

Brené Brown found that no one wants to talk about shame, and "the more you don't want to talk about it, the more you have it."[18] So the first step in getting at it is to stop repressing shame by bringing it out into the light of day. To repeat, awareness is the first step in changing the way our brain is wired. The following quiz helps identify your shame-driven thoughts and behaviors. It provides a set of statements on the way you relate to people and events. Check off any of the items that come close to being true for you.

After taking the quiz, look it over. Each of these statements reflects shame-based thinking, beliefs, and behaviors. It doesn't matter how many you checked. What matters is looking deeper into the items you have checked and becoming more aware of the ways in which this condition shows up in your life and thwarts you as a person. Take your time with this. Don't judge or condemn yourself; that's just shame coming through the back door. Let go of any judgments and simply become aware of how shame happens in you. See what beliefs are at the bottom of it. Then gradually see how this condition might change. What if you didn't believe that thought, see things that way, or behave in that manner? The more awareness you gain from exploring your pattern, the closer you come to changing the condition.

Empowering Your Upside

So far we've been focused on the downside of shame, which is a life of debilitating stress, diminished higher-brain function, and unrealized dreams. Let's shift to the upside, where peace, joy, well-being, and the realization of your full potential come into focus. This is the end of the stress that shame generates. You can start by taking

FRAGMENTATION QUIZ

○ I often think what I do is not quite good enough.

○ I resist feeling "bad" emotions in an effort to be "good," but find that "bad" emotions occasionally take hold of me.

○ I view emotionality as a sign of weakness and a lack of control.

○ I'm afraid to question authority when I see a better way.

○ At work, it's necessary to act confident even when I'm not.

○ I project an image of a happy or secure person without really feeling it.

○ I have a tendency to withdraw when challenged.

○ I often put on a face to hide what I feel.

○ I care more about what others think of me than I'd like to admit.

○ I am generally restrained when it comes to emotional expression, but often have stronger feelings than I express.

○ I feel the need to defend myself.

○ I have a hard time feeling safe in an intimate relationship.

○ I sometimes shudder at something I've said.

○ At times, I cringe when I remember something I regret from the past.

○ I feel rejected when people disagree with me.

○ I tend to avoid eye contact with other people.

○ I find it difficult to receive gifts from others.

○ I feel like I am not as successful as I should be at this point in my life.

○ I try to win people's approval.

This worksheet is available for download at theendofstressbook.com/worksheets.

a simple first step toward minimizing the propensity of shame to diminish your better self. It involves quietly Acknowledging the Difference You Make each day, in all the ordinary and extraordinary ways you do. You've already practiced a version of this step. It's the process called Mark the Moment, but here you apply it to marking those occasions when what you have been or done has been "good enough" or more than "good enough."

Mark the Moment each and every time you notice something you did, large or small, that contributed positively to someone or some effort. It could be as large as leading a group to success and as seemingly small as making a child smile. And please include the difference you make in becoming better and better at choosing peace instead of stress. Allow yourself to experience the peace and satisfaction of a job well done, along with the elation over the progress you're making in growing the talent and strengths you possess. Mark those moments by stopping to tell yourself that this accomplishment is important.

The Strengths-Finding Tool

There is another tool that helps pull your upside to the forefront. It's called the Strengths-Finding Tool, and it provides a basic inventory of your strengths. It offers a kind of repertoire of your intangible personal assets. In addition, it helps you focus on identifying and then accentuating what is right about you, meaning your strengths and talents, which is an antidote to all that shame says is wrong with you. Take your time. My guess is that if you allow yourself to feel your personal strengths as you check each one, by the end of the inventory you will feel relatively stress free.

Check any of the strengths listed below that you possess. It doesn't matter if you don't currently use it; it's still a strength, so check it. Take your time with this. One you've selected all the items that pertain to you, go back over the list. Reflect on each item that describes you. If it's an item you use, recall how and where. Consider how you might increase this strength. If it's an item you don't use, think of how you might put it to work.

This tool is not something you do once and then file away. It's something to keep in front of you as you go through your day to remind you to notice when you're using a particular strength or exhibiting a particular personal quality. Using the Strengths-Finding Tool—and Acknowledging the Difference You Make when you do something well—are forms of cognitive retraining that counter the shame-based voice in your head that says you're not good enough. It works to change how you relate to and experience yourself. As you now know, a change in experience changes your brain. In this case, it activates the neuroplasticity that rewires you for greater self-esteem instead of an ongoing barrage of shame. Making a practice of identifying and acknowledging your strengths is vitally important. It will lower your stress level. On the other hand, living with shame will promote a condition of chronic stress.

Also expand on the list of items on the Strengths-Finding Tool. The tool is meant to prime the pump, so build on it. As you go through the day and discover a strength or quality in you that isn't on the list, note it.

When you reflect on your strengths, think broadly. There are strengths that reveal themselves in roles you play, such as being a parent, coaching a team, teaching Sunday school, gardening, or volunteering at a charity. There are also personality strengths, such as being humorous or openhearted. There are interpersonal strengths that make you great at relationships, such as being a good listener. There are aptitudes you possess, such as being artistic or mechanical or good at science and math, or having a green thumb or a passion for history. There are social skills that make you a good communicator and business skills that enable you to contribute to a mission.

STRENGTHS-FINDING TOOL

General Strengths	Analytical Strengths
Are you:	**Are you:**
O Social	O Organized
O Artistic	O Systematic
O Intellectual	O Methodical
O Mechanical	O Logical
O Athletic	O Detail oriented
O Spiritual	O Prudent
O An outdoors person	O Deductive/insightful
Innovative Strengths	**Social Strengths**
Are you:	**Are you:**
O Creative	O Open-minded
O Original	O Supportive
O Imaginative	O Astute
O Inventive	O Hospitable

STRENGTHS-FINDING TOOL *(cont'd from pg 147)*

Innovative Strengths *(cont'd)*	Social Strengths *(cont'd)*
Are you:	**Are you:**
O Daring	O Kindhearted
O Intuitive	O Gregarious
O Curious	O Empathetic
O Insightful	O Inclusive
O Sensitive	O Tolerant
O Visionary	O A good listener
Entrepreneurial Strengths	**Work Strengths**
Are you:	**Are you:**
O An avid learner	O Cooperative
O Assertive	O Decisive
O Pragmatic	O Efficient
O Persuasive	O Focused
O Enthusiastic	O Fair

STRENGTHS-FINDING TOOL *(cont'd)*

Entrepreneurial Strengths *(cont'd)*	Work Strengths *(cont'd)*
Are you:	**Are you:**
O Energetic	O Motivated
Spiritual Strengths	**Emotional Strengths**
Are you:	**Are you:**
O Loving	O Self-aware
O Peaceful	O Balanced
O Present	O Motivated
O Authentic	O Caring
O Forgiving	O Enthusiastic
O Appreciative	O Happy
O Accepting/ nonjudgmental	O Humorous

The range of strengths is broad, so as you step into this process of strength-finding, think broadly.

And, as I said in the instruction, don't omit the strengths you are not currently using; they're still strengths. For example, if someone is good at illustrating but hasn't drawn a picture in a while, it is still an artistic strength they possess and could develop further. It is also a strength if other people have more of it, or are better at it than you. For example, Whoopi Goldberg's strength as an actress is not nullified by the accomplishments of Meryl Streep. It's also a strength if you sometimes misuse it, such as having a good sense of humor that sometimes bites or turns sarcastic.

As you do the strength inventory, as well as acknowledging the difference you make, you might encounter a voice in your head telling you it's conceited to focus on your strengths. Or that it demonstrates a lack of humility to acknowledge the difference you make. It's quite the opposite. Genuinely affirming something good and true about yourself actually humbles you, and the very heart of humility is gratitude. So see this tool as a means for extending gratitude for the gifts you've been given and for the difference you make. You can even add your gratitude for your gifts to your weekly practice of counting your blessings. We have the responsibility to grow and extend the gifts we possess, and acknowledging them is part of what makes them grow. When shame raises its ugly, critical head, use the Thought Awareness Tool to bring these negating, cynical thoughts into awareness, and choose not to believe what they say. Then see what happens to your stress level.

The Fully Functioning Person

Overcoming shame is an essential part of becoming a fully functioning, whole person. Let me summarize what Carl Rogers said about becoming whole. He said it begins with accepting yourself, exactly as you are. It's closing the gap between your ideal self and your real self; the gap between the person you think you should be and who you actually are at the moment. This entails being mindful of the times when you are acting as though you were something that you are not. It's becoming increasingly aware of the facades and pretenses you're running and letting them go. It's coming to understand that it really doesn't help to act one way when you feel another way. It doesn't help to act as though you know the answers when you don't. Being open to your experience is essential to personality change, and this includes being open to feelings. The more you are able to experience all of your feelings, the less you're afraid of any of your feelings, including shame. This enables you to detect and correct mistakes, see misperceptions and let them go, and identify and change negative behaviors. Rogers found that the more you trust your experience, the more your experience becomes your authority.[19] Other people's ideas and judgments, while taken into account, cease to overrule you. It's as Alan Watts said, "When a man no longer confuses himself with the definition that others have given him, he is at once universal and unique."[20]

Because of your openness, you are able to be less judgmental and more empathic with others—and yourself. Relationships become more meaningful, as opposed to how meaningless they feel when two shame-based minds hide behind facades. You can accept that you're not perfect, that you don't always function in the way that you would like to function or achieve the result you'd like to see. No one does. But through this understanding, you come to see that although you're not perfect, you are enough. It's a curious paradox that accepting yourself as you are, flaws, strengths, and all, is actually how you grow into a fully functioning person. Self-acceptance is essential in becoming stress free because it is the path that leads away from shame.

Below is a list of attributes of a whole person. Check three qualities on this list that you would like to strengthen, starting today. Once you have made progress with the attributes you've selected, you can return to this list and choose another one or more to work on.

Carl Rogers, who the National Institute of Mental Health determined was the most influential psychotherapist in America,[21] concluded from his enormous body of research that the core of

THE ATTRIBUTES OF A WHOLE PERSON

Check three qualities listed below that you want to strengthen.

O Spontaneous	O Creative, curious, and interested in learning
O Open to your own experience of life	O A good listener
O Able to experience all of your feelings	O Unconditionally loving
O Undefended and self-accepting	O Constructive in your responses
O The courage to be imperfect	O Collaborative and democratic
O Nonjudgmental with others	O Open to other people's ideas and points of view but not governed by them
O Living more completely in the moment	O Empathic and compassionate
O A clear sense of purpose	O Able to forgive
O Trusting your own judgment in finding your best available answer to any situation	O Able to give and receive appreciation and admiration
	O The capacity to retreat into the quiet of your own being

This worksheet is available for download at theendofstressbook.com/worksheets.

human nature is "exquisitely rational," "essentially positive," and "thoroughly trustworthy."[22] Rogers held you and your potential in high regard, perhaps higher than the way you see yourself. Rogers' view counts because it was informed by research, not shame.

Take a moment and consider that this exquisitely rational, essentially positive, and thoroughly trustworthy nature is in you. It's the core of the motherboard that nature embedded within you. The latent power of human nature is embedded in the neural circuitry of the brain. Put your hand on the top of your head for just a moment. Consider the fact that there are a hundred billion neurons pulsing in your brain, accomplishing everything from slipping the key into the car ignition to eliciting the left brain to capture the creative insight from the right brain and turn it into a work of art. A hundred billion neurons are the equivalent of the number of stars that populate the Milky Way. The next time you're out in nature on a clear night, look up at the Milky Way and realize that this unending array of twinkling light represents what is contained inside your skull. Then consider that there are as many as ten thousand synapses connecting neurons, one to another, in a vast system of networks. Put it all together, and you have an astronomical value that approximates the infinite. Take a moment and imagine how powerful this system can make you. The evidence of it is exhibited in museums around the world. It also gives us the capacity to love, connect, and create community. It drives us to contribute to the greater good, and, properly trained, it attains enlightenment. And that's just a thumbnail sketch of what it can do.

At the end of this chapter is a worksheet called The Whole Brain. It lists brain functions that empower a fully functioning human being. These attributes represent a vibrant, emotionally positive, and stress-free brain that enables you to succeed at life.[23] Look this list over. As you do, check off those attributes you would like to develop or increase. Your brain is waiting on neuroplastic processes to wake up your innate power. Those neuroplastic processes are, in turn, waiting for a change in mind-set; and that change in mind-set is wait-ing on you.

Your Practice This Week

- Become more and more aware of the difference you make and out-comes you accomplish each day this week. Mark those moments by taking time out to experience the joy and satisfaction they produce.
- Use the Strengths-Finding Tool to increase your awareness of your strengths and talents. Work with it each day, adding other strengths and qualities you possess that are not on the list.
- Accentuate each of the qualities you checked from the Attributes of a Whole Person checklist.

And Keep Practicing the Following

- Remember to use the Three Sane Choices Tool if you find yourself feeling powerless in a situation and Feel It to Heal It if you find tension mounting in your body.
- Practice the Thirty-Second Time-Out for Peace a few times each day.
- Continue using the Getting Clear Tool once every day (twice a day is even better).
- Use the Clear Button Tool to clear a stress-provoking pattern of thinking.
- Continue using the Thought Awareness Tool.
- Continue starting your day in quiet. Take breaks and go for walks in a green setting. If you have a difficult problem, sleep on it and in the morning see whether there is an answer to it that your brain dreamed up. Once a week, count your blessings.

Tools

YOUR WHOLE BRAIN
Check the attributes you want to grow
○ **Executive functions,** increasing your proficiency at planning, strategizing, decision making, abstract thinking, cognitive flexibility, error detection, and goal-directed action
○ **Creative processes,** where the dots start connecting themselves, turning creative insight into tangible innovation
○ **Emotional regulation,** where you feel vibrant and inspired, but not so emotionally charged that you become manic, chaotic, or rigid
○ **The condition of learning** facilitated by attention, memory, and curiosity working in concert
○ **The passion and motivation** to persist in the pursuit of a significant goal
○ **The capacity to extinguish fear** and quiet fight/flight/freeze reactions to attain the fearless self-confidence that adversity does not unsettle
○ **The response flexibility** that neutralizes rash impulses, signaling you to pause and reflect before acting in an aggressive or defensive manner
○ **The altruism** that enables you to move beyond limited self-interest and think and act for the larger good
○ **The attuned communication** that achieves interpersonal resonance
○ **The empathy** that enables you to see, feel, and understand a situation from someone else's point of view
○ **The parental love** that raises healthy children
○ **The romantic love** and sexual passion that sustain intimacy
○ **The insight** that produces the autobiographical memories to relate the past to the present, so you can guide the future
○ **The intuition** to discern the solution to a problem that eludes the intellect
○ **The holism** that achieves the congruency between thought, belief, intention, and action to sustain personal integrity

➤ **This worksheet is available for download at theendofstressbook.com/worksheets.**

12

The Blue Zone of Connection

In his book *The Blue Zones*, Dan Buettner takes us into communities around the world where people live unusually long lives—and profoundly happy, healthy, and much less stressful ones. One such zone is the Greek island of Ikaria, where Buettner and his research team spent more than a year studying the island's centenarians. In the chapter entitled "The Greek Blue Zone," Buettner tells the story of a Greek war veteran named Stamatis, who emigrated from Ikaria to the United States after World War II. His arm had been mangled from a combat wound, and he came to the States in hopes of medical treatment that might repair it. He settled on Long Island, married a Greek-American woman, had children, and eventually achieved the American dream.

Then, in his midsixties, Stamatis was diagnosed with lungcancer and given nine months to live. Instead of undergoing aggressive cancer treatment, Stamatis decided to return home to Ikaria. He wanted to die in his native land among his native people and be buried with his ancestors in the cemetery overlooking the Aegean Sea. But once Stamatis was back in the bosom of village life, something completely unexpected, if not miraculous, began to unfold. The loving care he received from his mother and wife improved his condition and he began to feel better. His heart began to open, and he felt inspired in ways he hadn't felt in decades. It's common for a life-threatening illness to turn our eyes to heaven, and so it was with Stamatis. He returned to the Greek Orthodox faith in which he had been raised, and on Sundays he visited the grave of his grandfather, who had once been the community's priest. He gradually recovered his strength, which gave him the energy to reconnect with his childhood friends to the point that nearly every afternoon he went out with friends. They drank wine, shared and laughed at each other's stories and banter, and played board games. He eventually felt strong enough to plant a garden and even tend to the family vineyard, although he didn't expect to be around for the harvest. Nine months came and went, but he didn't die as medical statistics had predicted. Then more than thirty years passed. Instead of friends and family placing flowers on Stamatis's grave, they were toasting him on his hundredth birthday.[1]

What accounts for this miraculous outcome? There is a direct correlation between how long you will live and the quality of your connection to other people. Cultivating positive relationships that instill a sense of connectedness and belonging is literally how our organism thrives. It's a big part of what alleviates stress and prevents toxic stress hormones from ruining our cardiovascular system, dampening our immune system, and prematurely aging us. What happened to Stamatis of Ikaria is not an anomaly. The first study to reveal the biological connection between the quality of our interpersonal connections, our health, and how long we live was the Roseto Study. It has come to be called the Roseto Effect.

More than forty years ago, medical researchers were stumped by a bewildering statistic in the village of Roseto, Pennsylvania. Rosetans were nearly immune to the number-one cause of death in America—heart disease. Cardiac mortality rises with age, but not in Roseto. It dropped to near zero for men aged fifty-five to sixty-four. For men over sixty-five, the local death rate was half the national average. This made no medical sense, given that most of the men smoked, drank heavily, ate a high-fat diet, were poor, and did hard, backbreaking work in a rock quarry.

A team of medical researchers from Oklahoma University descended on the village to try to find out why. They pulled death certificates, performed physical exams, and conducted extensive interviews with villagers. But they could find no biological, genetic, environmental, or any other physical source to explain Rosetans' resistance to heart disease—until they stumbled across two social factors. First, they discovered that the crime rate in the village was *zero*. Second, they found that although the village was poor, no one was on public welfare.[2]

When they dug deeper, the researchers found that the family structure in Roseto was close-knit. Nearly all the homes contained three generations, and elders were held in high regard. Mealtimes were much more than a matter of eating; they were family time. Community events were also common in Roseto. In warm weather, neighbors took evening strolls and dropped in to visit one another. Sociologist John Bruhn of the University of Texas, who later coauthored a book about the village, said that Rosetans "radiated a kind of joyous team spirit as they celebrated religious festivals and family landmarks. Their social focus was on the family . . ."[3]

The researchers finally concluded that the village's immunity to heart disease and early death was the result of the strong sense of belonging that people felt. But sadly, the effect didn't last. The children of Roseto went off to college in pursuit of the American dream, and after graduation most of them moved to the big city, where the high-paying jobs were. As a result, the community gradually lost its cohesion, and in 1971 the village recorded its first death of a person under the age of forty-five from coronary disease. It went downhill from there. The traditional communal experience that enabled people to live longer, healthier lives eroded. The death rate eventually rose to the national average.[4]

In the ensuing forty years, scores of other studies have corroborated the Roseto Effect. In a recent review of 148 separate studies involving a combined 308,849 participants, it was found that people who cultivate strong relationships with friends, family, neighbors, and coworkers improve their odds of survival by 50 percent.[5] As I've said several times, stress is fear. Biologically, some form of fear must be present to excite a stress reaction. Love quiets fear. It's an antidote to the toxic stress hormones that can kill us. This is the key to why Stamatis of Ikaria is still drinking wine and playing dominos into the night. Conversely, the risk of death for people without strong social ties is quite high. It's comparable to smoking fifteen cigarettes a day, it's the equivalent to being an alcoholic, and it causes more health problems than being obese or failing to exercise.[6]

The happy and longer-than-expected life spans of Stamatis of Ikaria and the people of Roseto begs a question: how do you connect and stay connected? Fundamentally, sustaining our connection to others involves overcoming two major obstacles that typically and unwittingly undermine our intentions to connect. The first obstacle is our tendency to judge other people. Much of this is driven by the shame we feel that, as we saw in the last chapter, becomes too painful for the mind to hold. When that happens, our shame often projects its self-condemnation onto other people in the form of unkind judgments. The price we pay is separation. The second obstacle to connection is our unwillingness to forgive.

The Tendency to Judge

Most of us believe that our thoughts, even if they are critical, don't harm others as long as they remain in the private sanctum of our head. We think others can't sense the judgments we project or the condemnation we feel toward them. Well, think again; it's not the case. Our facial expression, body language, physical energy, emotional affect, stammers, stutters, and tics register in the other person's brain, betraying our attempts to conceal the judgments we're making. Equally, the range of cues our brain produces when we feel warmth and esteem also registers in the other person's brain. It's almost like we're able to read each other's minds. Actually, our brains are reading each other's minds.

The brain system that registers and reads these subtle cues is called the mirror neuron system. Mirror neurons track emotions, body language, tone of voice, and even another's unspoken intentions. When someone we know smiles at us or smirks, it literally sends a reverberation that oscillates throughout our brain. Their voice can animate their words with a tone that enables our brain to instantly understand their meaning, even if it's quite subtle. Somehow our brain gets the meaning without the other person having to explain anything.

Mirror neurons explain instant rapport and instant disdain. It's how Rodgers and Hammerstein were able to play off one another in creating beautiful harmonies. It's why, biologically, friends are healing and enemies are toxic, why hostility raises blood pressure and kindness lowers it, and why a dad's heavy footsteps coming up the front steps at the end of a stressful day stresses his children. "I know when my mom has a bad day," one child told a researcher studying kids and stress. "Because when she picks me up from after school she doesn't smile. She has a really frustrated look on her face."[7]

This child speaks for a lot of kids. A survey by the American Psychology Association found that 91 percent of children say what stresses them most is how stressed their parents have become.[8] Their mirror neurons mimic their parents' stress, and this causes children pernicious stress reactions. When we see someone suffering or in pain, mirror neurons actually make us feel their suffering or the pain.[9] It explains why hypochondriacs and medical students experience other people's symptoms even though they don't have the disease.

Basically, mirror neurons are copycats. They imitate the physical gestures, expressions, and behaviors of the other person. The identical cluster of mirror neurons that fired in your lover's brain when he or she smiled at you also fire inside your brain. Marco Iacoboni of UCLA School of Medicine writes, "The relatively simple physiological properties of mirror neurons allow us to understand the mental states of other people and practically puts us in another person's mind."[10]

Iacoboni deciphered the way mirror neurons process information to generate empathic understanding. He conducted an experiment in which he tracked the brain activity of subjects while they were viewing or mimicking pictures of faces that expressed the basic range of human emotion. He found that empathy was produced along a direct neural pathway from mirror neurons through to the insula and finally to the emotional brain.[11] The mirror neuron system sends a signal to the insula: a network that plays an important role in generating self-awareness and interpersonal experience, as well as mediating the experience of fear, surprise, sadness, anger, disgust, and happiness. The insula, in turn, sends the signal down to the emotional brain, where the signal is translated into emotion. The result is that you feel the feeling of the other person. Your lover's smile is translated into joy, their frown into sadness.

The Mirror Neuron–Empathy Test Drive

You can directly experience how mirror neurons generate empathy in you by watching the *Empathy Video*. This video presents a slide show that screens a number of photographs, one at a time. The images are of people's faces expressing the basic range of human emotions, from fear to happiness. Each photograph remains on screen for ten seconds before transitioning to the next one. Your task is to look at the face and sense the emotion the face is expressing. Allow yourself to feel the emotion on that face. See if you can enter that person's experience completely, as if it were your own experience. Be sensitive to your visceral responses, such as the sensation of your heart opening, the stirring of gut feelings, emotional contagion, and the state of your brain. As you read each face, don't analyze the expression. Just look at the face and wait for a feeling to come up in you. There is an old Zen saying that goes: *No need to figure anything out when you can feel your way through it.* If at any point during the slide show your mind wanders off, gently bring it back to the task.

You are likely to be surprised by how much empathy you are capable of feeling for another human being. So, right now, watch the *Empathy Video* by either scanning the QR code below or following the link below.

 Empathy Video Stream:
A four-and-a-half-minute stream of the *Empathy Video*.

https://www.youtube.com/watch?v=l1TURJp1rUk&feature =youtu.be

Empathy

Mirror neurons generate empathy, which is the opposite experience of judging and condemning. Empathy is significantly correlated with self-esteem, the opposite of shame.[12] Empathy is also the underlying foundation of social intelligence that determines how long we live.

Carl Rogers defined empathy as the willingness to enter another person's private world so completely that you lose all desire to judge them. He said, "We think we listen, but very rarely do we listen with real understanding, true empathy. Yet listening, of this very special kind, is one of the most potent forces for change in a relationship that I know."[13]

Being empathic with another person means that you temporarily lay aside your views and values in order to enter another's world without prejudice. Empathy involves being sensitive to whatever the other person is experiencing moment to moment. It includes communicating what you're sensing as you listen, without imposing it, and always being guided by the responses you receive from the other person.[14] But it is also an "as if" way of relating: as if I were hurting or frightened or elated in the same way this person is at present. Obviously, you are not the other person, and this "as-if" quality enables you to enter their experience without getting lost in it.

Empathy is a form of respect that makes relationships work at home, with friends, and even in business. Former CEO of Motorola, Bob Galvin, in speaking about his father, Paul, who founded Motorola, said, "My father once looked down at an assembly line of women and thought, *These ladies are all like my own mom—they have kids, homes to take care of, people who need them.* It motivated my father to work hard to give these women a better life because he saw his mother in all of them. . . . That's how it all begins—with fundamental respect and empathy."[15]

The path to positive relationships is mercifully simple, even if we tend to botch it. It can be summed up in four rules. The first three rules we have covered:

Listen better, with empathy. Judge less. Love unconditionally.

These three are about being more loving, if for no other reason than the fact that love is the way our biology functions best. And here is another fact. We fail at love more than we may care to admit. We fail at empathy and acceptance, especially when stressed and afraid. At those times, the state of our brain makes us capable of serious mistakes, reacting in regrettable ways that can be hurtful, harmful, and at times destructive.

This is where the fourth rule comes into play, which is to forgive more. If our health and longevity depend on our capacity to love, which they do, then forgiveness is a biological imperative. So, let's turn to the second obstacle to connection, which is an unwillingness to forgive.

An Unwillingness to Forgive

The second obstacle to sustaining meaningful connections is our unwillingness to forgive someone for the pain they caused us. More often than not, our unwillingness stems from a need to protect ourselves from further harm, or to punish another person for the pain they've inflicted (or both.) Although these feelings may be justified, nonetheless they prolong a state of fear and enmity that amplifies the stress gene, activating the brain's fear center to flood us with painful emotional memories. It can affect the way we relate to people generally, making us reticent to trust and open up in ways that deepen a connection.

Without forgiveness there can be no release or reconciliation. When we don't forgive mistakes, we perpetuate guilt and shame, and we become imprisoned in conflict, stress, and separation. This moves us in the opposite direction from cultivating relationships that foster a happy, healthy, long, and stress-free life. Given that forgiveness is a biological necessity, it's critical that we consider why it is we don't forgive so we can move past it.

Why We Don't Forgive

At the top of the list is the belief that not forgiving somehow protects us. But this is a delusion. An unwillingness to forgive is tantamount to taking poison and expecting the other person to die. Biologically, forgiveness is the antidote to the poison.

Another reason we don't forgive is our fear that forgiving opens the door to being hurt again. Forgiving doesn't require that we reconnect with an irresponsible or mean-spirited person. We also refuse to forgive because we think that forgiving condones the act, but forgiveness has never been about condoning bad or destructive behavior.

Often, we refuse to forgive because we believe the person who injured us deserves our anger and should be condemned and punished. We might even see forgiving as handing the offending person a free pass to fail us or hurt us all over again. But it just might be the case that the people we can't forgive have changed. They may have learned from their mistakes, and they may even be sorry. Our unwillingness to forgive locks us into perceiving them through the eyes of the past instead of seeing who they may have become.

We can even delude ourselves into thinking our unwillingness to forgive maintains our control over the injuring party. In truth, the refusal to forgive is a painful state of mind that controls us, stresses us, and keeps us stuck in the past.

The Forgiveness Tool

Forgiveness isn't necessarily a once-and-for-all-time event. Often, it's a one-day-at-a-time process in which you gradually let go of the hurt and reclaim your peace of mind by making it more important than the grievance. There is a tool that can help as you move through this process. It begins with bringing to mind a person who has been difficult for you to forgive. You allow yourself to feel the pain this person caused you. You feel how difficult it is for you to forgive what they did.

Next you make the effort to perceive the humanity in this person somewhere: a little gleam emanating from them that perhaps you haven't been able to see. This can be difficult at first, but it's worth getting past the resistance, if only for the duration of this exercise. Look until you see some trace of brightness shining through the painful picture that you hold of this person, softening the picture, making this person appear somewhat brighter, with the potential for a kinder heart than the grievance allows you to see.

Then silently recite the following words, directing them to this person. *I forgive you. I release you to your highest good. I free myself from this grievance and all the pain that has come from it. I release the present from the past and free my future.*

You repeat the words a second time, and when you're finished, you let this person fade from mind and disappear. As the person fades into the background, imagine that you have come into full view, in sharp focus. See yourself as bright and vibrant and liberated from the pain of this past event.

Next, apply this same process to yourself to forgive a mistake or misdeed you committed, simply by making yourself the one in need of forgiveness.

We would all do well to remember that judging others and refusing to forgive are poor biological strategies. The scientific evidence makes the choice clear—it's a choice between a nonjudgmental, unconditionally accepting way of being with people and all the emotional and medical problems disconnection is bound to cause. There is no getting around it: When you judge and condemn, you turn up the stress gene, and your brain floods your system with stress hormones. Cells move toward the overexpression of proinflammatory molecules that age you prematurely and the underexpression of all the immune-boosting systems that produce antibodies and antivirals. Who, in their right mind, wants that?

Creating positive relationships is not as complex as we sometimes make it. When you find yourself in disagreement with someone you love, ask yourself this basic question: *Do I want to be right or do I want to be connected?* See what happens to the stress and dissonance when you let go of the need to be right and are willing to see someone else's point of view or validate someone else's experience.

Your Practice This Week

- Call a friend or family member you've meant to connect with but have kept putting off. Make a date to get together.
- Take the mirror neuron / empathy test drive by watching the *Empathy Video*. Follow the instructions given on screen.
- Do the forgiveness exercise to clear a grievance you have with someone else. Then apply this same process to yourself to forgive a mistake or misdeed you committed, by making yourself the one in need of forgiveness.

And Keep Practicing the Following

- Remember to use the Three Sane Choices Tool if you find yourself feeling powerless in a situation and Feel It to Heal It if you find tension mounting in your body.
- Practice Acknowledging the Difference You Make by becoming aware of the positive impacts you have upon others, and various large and small ways you've made a positive impact each day this week.
- Accentuate each of the qualities you checked from the Attributes of a Whole Person checklist.
- Practice the Thirty-Second Time-Out for Peace Tool a few times each day.
- Continue using the Getting Clear Tool once every day (twice a day is even better).
- Use the Clear Button Tool to clear a stress-provoking pattern of thinking.
- Continue using the Thought Awareness Tool.

- Continue starting your day in quiet. Take breaks and go for walks in a green setting. If you have a difficult problem, sleep on it and in the morning see whether there is an answer to it that your brain dreamed up. Once a week, count your blessings.

Tools

The Positive Relationship Tool

- Listen better, with empathy.
- Judge less.
- Love unconditionally.
- Forgive more.

The Forgiveness Tool

- Bring to mind a person who is difficult for you to forgive.
- Feel the pain this person caused you and perhaps others. Feel how difficult it is for you to forgive what they did.
- I am going to invite you to do something that may be difficult, but allow yourself to go with the process for a moment. Approach this exercise as you would an experiment, with an interest in seeing what might happen.
- I invite you to perceive the humanity in this person somewhere: a little gleam emanating from them that perhaps you haven't been able to see.
- Look until you see some trace of brightness shining through the painful picture you hold of this person, softening the picture, making this person appear somewhat brighter, with the potential for a kinder heart than the grievance allows you to see.
- Now silently recite the words below, directing the words to this person.

I forgive you.
I release you to your highest good.

I free myself from this grievance and all the pain that has come from it.

I release the present from the past and free my future.

- Say these words one more time.
- When you finish, see this person fade and disappear from view.
- As this person fades into the background, imagine that you have come into full view, in sharp focus. See yourself as bright and vibrant. See yourself as liberated from the pain of this past event.

Forgiving Myself Tool

- Bring to mind a mistake you made that has been difficult for you to forgive.
- Feel the pain of your regret.
- Perceive the humanity in yourself: a little gleam emanating from you that perhaps you have been unable to see because of the mistake.
- See some trace of brightness shining through the painful picture you hold of yourself, softening the picture, making you appear somewhat brighter.
- Now silently recite the words below.

I forgive myself.

I release myself to my highest good.

I free myself from this grievance and all the pain that has come from it.

I release the present from the past and free my future.

Forgiveness Process Audio:
A six-minute audio in which Don walks you through the Forgiveness process.

http://www.beyondword.com/theendofstress/tag11_Forgiveness.mp3

Forgiving Myself Process Audio:
A six-minute audio in which Don walks you through the process of forgiving yourself.

http://www.beyondword.com/theendofstress/tag12_Forgiving-Myself.mp3

13

The Power of Suggestion: You Get What You Expect to Get

Rubbing a rabbit's foot, crossing your fingers, knocking on wood, or wishing on a falling star all have one thing in common—the power of suggestion. The magic you imagine in the bones and fur of the rabbit's foot makes you feel lucky and hopeful, which invites into your mind the anticipation that an outcome you desire could actually happen.

Does that sound silly to you? It might, but the scientific evidence suggests that your anticipation mobilizes vast inner resources and directs those resources toward fulfilling your desire. Irving Kirsch of Harvard Medical School and Maryanne Garry of Victoria University of Wellington teamed up to review the most recent and intriguing effects of the power of suggestion on cognition and behavior.[1] The evidence shows once you anticipate that a desired outcome could happen, you set in motion a chain of thoughts and actions that work together to actually make it happen. "The effects of suggestion," Dr. Garry states, "are wider and often more surprising than many people might otherwise think. If we can harness the power of suggestion," Garry concludes, "we can improve people's lives."[2]

The power of suggestion appears to be at the center of why some people succeed at school, business, or athletics while others fail, and why some people's illness or pain resolves and others' gets worse. Suggestion has the power to improve your performance in a challenging situation, like giving a speech or taking a test. It causes placebos to relieve pain or reduce symptoms. It can even improve eyesight, generate weight loss, reverse the aging process, and change the course of a life-threatening disease.

No one outside of Hollywood is suggesting that you can become Superman or Wonder Woman. There are limits imposed on your cognitive and physical abilities. But these findings make it clear that the popular conception of those limits needs a major revision. It's quite clear from a number of studies that believing you are limited or blocked in some way drives the limitation. The great martial artist Bruce Lee said, "There are no limits. There are only plateaus, and you must not stay there. You must go beyond them."[3]

Evidence is accumulating to suggest that our very thoughts are capable of extending cognitive and physical limits beyond anything science would have predicted. It appears that the limits we perceive are not necessarily set by nature, but by our own mental attitude.

The Placebo Effect

The placebo effect describes real psychological and physiological changes that occur when the mind has been tricked into expecting a medical intervention to succeed, such as a pill or injection, when in fact the substance is inert. In itself, the placebo does nothing; it's the mind that generates the beneficial effect. The classic study of the placebo effect was of saline injections that significantly reduced the pain of badly wounded soldiers who were told that the injections contained a powerful opiate.[4] That study was the first to make clear that pain has more to do with the mind than the severity of a physical injury. While the majority of research on the placebo effect has focused on medical issues, there is growing evidence of placebo effects in other areas.

One such study relates to prospective memory. Prospective memory is how the brain remembers details or events that are to occur in the future. It gets us to appointments on time, helps us pay our bills when they are due, enables us to follow a recipe in preparing a meal, anticipates the next steps in a strategic plan, and reminds us to take medication at required intervals. We couldn't get through life without prospective memory.

Chronic stress debilitates prospective memory, and researchers at Victoria University wanted to see if it was possible to enhance it with a placebo. They set up a study in which the researchers went to great lengths to convince subjects that a placebo they'd been given was a powerful "smart drug" that improved cognitive function and memory. In fact, the so-called smart drug was nothing more than vitamin C powder mixed with water. One group received the placebo and one group didn't. Then the researchers put both groups through a high-effort prospective memory task. Prospective memory improved in the group that had ingested the vitamin C placebo, while the group that didn't receive the placebo showed no improvement. The group whose minds had been tricked into *anticipating* cognitive improvement actually achieved it.[5]

In another study on placebos and memory, subjects were told that a certain odor would improve implicit memory. Implicit memory is unconscious. It represents information you retrieve in an effortless, automatic manner. It is how your fingers find the letters on your keyboard without your thinking about it, and why you never forget how to ride a bike. When the subjects in this study were exposed to the odor, implicit memory actually responded faster and demonstrated stronger cuing.[6]

The power of anticipation also works to enhance athletic performance. In recent years athletes have used performance-enhancing drugs to expand the limits of their talent. Yet research suggests that much of the benefit derived from these drugs may not come from the compound itself but from the athletes' expectancy—their belief that the drug will elevate performance. In a study conducted by the Scottish Institute of Sport, sixteen athletes competing in a series of one-thousand-meter time trials were administered baking soda mixed with placebo additives and told that the cocktail was a performance-enhancing steroid. Simply believing they were on steroids improved their performance. In contrast, athletes who were administered a real performance-enhancing drug without knowing it yielded no significant improvement.[7]

The Research of Ellen Langer

Perhaps nothing has turned our limited view of human potential on its head more than the research of Ellen Langer of Harvard University. Recall the first exercise you did as you embarked on this book's journey. It was a guided process based on a quote from William James, the father of American psychology, who said, "If you can change your mind, you can change your life." He said, "Belief creates the actual fact." One way to reinforce a belief is to visualize that belief coming true. So in that guided process you invoked the belief that you could generate a real breakthrough with stress and anxiety.

Well, Ellen Langer's research proves that what William James asserted more than a hundred years ago is true. She's shown that mind over matter is real. In this book, you've learned that a positive change of mind changes your brain, not only to end stress, but also to expand higher-brain function. Langer has found that we can even use our minds to trick our bodies into turning back the clock. As you read the following accounts of how people stretched their capacity, think back to the quote from William James and reassert your belief that you can attain and sustain a stress-free life.

In 1979, Langer conducted perhaps her most famous experiment, with men in their late seventies and early eighties, who were languishing in nursing homes.[8] She took the men on a one-week retreat during which they pretended it was 1959. It was as if they were in a play. They wore clothes that were fashionable in 1959, ate the food they ate then, carried photo IDs of how they looked in that year, and were encouraged to behave as they had twenty years before. They were even given newspapers and magazines from 1959 to read and shown films and television programs from 1959.

The results were astonishing. Compared to the control group, which went on an ordinary retreat, the time travelers showed greater improvements in joint flexibility and manual dexterity. Their arthritis began to retreat, and their IQs improved.

I related this study to my friend Kay, whose ninety-one-year-old mother lives with her. That night, Kay offered her mother a piece of dark chocolate. Her mother asked how much it had cost. "Only about two dollars," Kay said. Her mother was shocked at the amount. "*Two dollars!*" she said. "I can't believe a bar of chocolate costs that much."

"The cost is not that much," Kay said. "You can hardly buy anything for two dollars."

"Yes, of course," her mother acknowledged after thinking about it. "I guess my mind is still back in the 1950s." Kay said that normally she would have laughed at her mom, but not after learning about Ellen Langer's study. This time she didn't shrug her mother off or become annoyed with her mother's misplaced sense of what things should cost. Kay used the occasion to get her mother to open up about the good old days when things were cheaper. She asked her mom what life was like during that decade, and that night her mother told her all about it. There was a visibly positive effect from making space for her to reminisce. At the end of the evening, Kay said her mother looked years younger, and that night her mother slept better than she had in a long time. She had traveled back in time, and somehow her biological state had gone with her, just like the elderly men in Langer's study.

Recently an eighty-year-old friend of mine told her doctor she was having trouble retrieving words. The issue sometimes meant that she couldn't complete a thought in conversing with someone. Her doctor said it was normal for someone her age, but she didn't settle for that. She insisted on a referral and went to a neuropsychologist, who put her into an aggressive program to strengthen her memory. She's making real progress, and it's helped her confidence and self-esteem. All too often, seniors are treated as "over the hill" without any understanding that treating them this way is what creates the condition.

Langer also conducted a study with hotel workers who clean rooms.[9] These workers are typically assigned fifteen rooms a day and spend half an hour cleaning each room, an effort that exceeds the level of daily exercise the surgeon general prescribes. But the workers thought their job didn't qualify as exercise, and since they were too tired at the end of their shift to go to the gym, they believed they weren't getting any exercise. Dr. Langer divided the hotel workers into two groups. In one group, she reinforced the mind-set that the physical exertion in their job achieved the recommended level of physical fitness. The second group was not given this information. After four weeks, without any change in diet or activity, people in the first group lost weight. Their body fat dropped, and even their blood pressure improved. The only thing that had changed was the group's mind-set. There was no improvement in the second group.

It may be hard to believe that a change in mind-set could actually improve eyesight as bad as 20/70 or even 20/160, yet it did.[10] It makes one wonder if we're all wearing mental blinders. The evidence shows that we are! This can change; it's a matter of respecting the latent power of our thoughts. In his memoir, Thomas Merton wrote what I believe gets to the heart of the problem: "Perhaps I am stronger than I think. Perhaps I am even afraid of my strength and turn it against myself, thus making myself weak."[11]

The strength Merton is referring to is as near to you as your own thoughts. Years ago, I knew a young man who mistakenly thought something that influenced the course of his cancer. In his mid-twenties, he was diagnosed with stage-2 adult Hodgkin's lymphoma. The cancer had been found early, but even so, his prognosis was considered highly unfavorable. Yet when his oncologist delivered the bad news, this young man somehow heard the opposite, and he left the clinic thinking the doctor had told him that his chances were *highly favorable*. During the course of his treatment, his mind-set was built on the anticipation that every step of his medical care was achieving the *highly favorable* result of complete remission, which is exactly what happened. It wasn't until his case was presented during the hospital's grand rounds by his oncologist that he realized he'd misunderstood. He said that had he known the verdict that medical statistics predicted, he probably would have died. He was absolutely certain that the mind-set his misunderstanding produced saved his life.

One of the oldest forms of suggestion is hypnosis, but for most of the last thirty years it was frowned upon by medical science. That has all changed. "There are studies that show that hypnosis is stronger than the placebo effect," David Spiegel of Stanford University School of Medicine says. "It's not mind over matter, but mind matters." Dr. Spiegel adds that three out of four adults can be hypnotized.[12]

Hypnosis is effective in helping people quit smoking, lose weight, and manage phobias and pain. Increasingly, surgical patients are opting for hypnosis in place of anesthesia. It's been shown to reduce the pain in something as excruciatingly painful as childbirth. One pregnant woman practiced self-hypnosis every night for three months, and when she went into labor, she was able to mentally block the pain.

Under hypnosis, patients can also be taught to shift from being afraid of something in the outside world to feeling calm in that situation by imaging a safe place, like a beach. For example, a person afraid of flying can be placed under hypnosis and desensitized to every aspect of air travel. Their mind-set changes from frightened and unable to manage stressful thoughts to feeling relaxed and more in control. The evidence for the power of suggestion has become so convincing that the National Institutes of Health is studying how it can be applied in pain management, and researchers at University of Washington at Seattle are studying to see if virtual reality–assisted hypnosis can reduce burn victims' anxiety and pain.

The Shaping Reality Tool

The proof is there. The power of your mind can shape your reality as you know it. Harness this power and you become the master of your fate. There is a simple tool called Shaping Reality that can generate the anticipation that drives the power of suggestion in order to end stress and achieve the health, wealth, and love you desire. Use this tool on a daily basis to amplify your expectancy for achieving success.*

Here's what you do: Get into a comfortable position and close your eyes. Select a current goal you wish to achieve. Imagine as clearly as you can this outcome as you want it to happen. Pretend that it has already come to pass, and see your life as it would exist at that moment. Let go of all restraints on your thinking and involve the sensory parts of your brain. Hear the sounds that are present when the outcome is realized. Smell the air and feel the temperature in the environment. Visualize what you will see. Broaden that with

---

* This tool is a modification of a tool created by my business partner, Kaarin Alisa, called Igniting the Blueprint.

colors, people, and anything else that's meaningful to you. Feel the feelings you imagine will overcome you when this outcome is realized. Make these desired feelings as strong as you can. If you are happy, allow them to place a smile on your face or make you laugh out loud. If you are relieved, let the relief lift your spirits. Let the emotions become real. Sustain these desired emotions for as long as you can, but for no more than a minute. As you conclude the exercise, let everything go. Have faith that you have now locked your internal guidance system on your desired outcome.

Your Practice This Week

Apply the power of suggestion through the Shaping Reality Tool to imagine a successful outcome to an important personal goal.

And Keep Practicing the Following

- Remember to use the Three Sane Choices Tool if you find yourself feeling powerless in a situation and Feel It to Heal It if you find tension mounting in your body.
- Practice Acknowledging the Difference You Make by becoming aware of the positive impacts you have on others each day this week, in large and small ways.
- Accentuate each of the qualities you checked from the Attributes of a Whole Person checklist.
- Practice the Thirty-Second Time-Out for Peace Tool a few times each day.
- Continue using the Getting Clear Tool once every day (twice a day is even better).
- Use the Clear Button Tool to clear a stress-provoking pattern of thinking.
- Continue using the Thought Awareness Tool.

- Continue starting your day in quiet. Take breaks and go for walks in a green setting. If you have a difficult problem, sleep on it and in the morning see whether there is an answer to it that your brain dreamed up. Once a week, count your blessings.

Tools

Shaping Reality Tool

- Get into a comfortable position and close your eyes.
- Select a current goal and state to yourself the outcome you wish to achieve.
- Imagine this outcome as you want it to happen. Pretend that it has already come to pass, and see your life as it would exist at that moment. Let go of all restraints on your thinking. Tell yourself it's all right to imagine anything, regardless of whether you think it's probable or even possible.
- Involve the sensory parts of your brain. Hear the sounds that are present when the outcome is realized. Smell the air and feel the temperature in the environment. Picture what you will see.
- Now see into the periphery of the picture. What elements of life are around you? Who is with you? Make the colors and elements of your imagined outcome vivid. If people are present, what are they saying to you? What are you saying to them?
- As you continue to experience the vivid picture you have created, feel the feelings you imagine will overcome you when this outcome is realized. Do you feel joy? Do you feel satisfaction? Do you feel relief from pain or fear? And as you imagine the feelings you will have, bring them close and actually feel them as if they are your experience, right here, right now.
- Make these desired feelings as strong as you can. If you are happy, allow them to place a smile on your face or make you laugh out

loud. If you are relieved, let the relief lift your spirits. Let the emotions become real.

- Sustain these desired emotions for as long as you can, but for no more than a minute.
- Then let everything go. Let go of the emotions and let go of the picture.
- You have now primed the pump of your thinking and emotional centers to lock your internal guidance system on your desired outcome.

The Shaping Reality Guided Process Audio:
A five-minute audio in which Don walks you through the Shaping Reality guided process.

http://www.beyondword.com/theendofstress/tag13_Shaping -Reality.mp3

SUSTAINING IT

Every Day in Every Way

14

Pulling It All Together

You've come a long way. You've learned a number of concepts and tools, and you have digested a lot of research on stress, peace, and the brain. The aim of this book has been to help you end stress. Peace, joy, and fulfillment begin where stress ends. Toward that purpose, this book has attempted to help you build a dynamically peaceful attitude and to teach you to apply this attitude every day, in whatever situations you have to face. In this chapter, we're going to pull everything together into a practical and simplified format that you can use to keep moving your life in this new, stress-free direction.

In an earlier chapter you worked at building a To-Be List to integrate with a set of external goals you delineated. The goal was to empower a clearer sense of inner purpose that would flow into whatever you were trying to achieve, thus mitigating stress and accentuating the power of peace. Following is a general To-Be List that directly relates to ways of being that facilitate positive neuroplasticity, quieting stress reactions and amplifying higher-brain function. I invite you to checkmark any of these ways of being that you want to accentuate with greater consistency.

TO-BE LIST

○ To be at peace

○ To be present here and now

○ To listen better

○ To judge less

○ To forgive more

○ To be empathic

○ To be grateful

○ To take time to stop and stand still

○ To allow creative insight

○ To let go of fear

○ To have faith in the face of adversity

○ To trust the process as it unfolds

○ To focus on the whole of life instead of the fragments

○ To rest in the quiet of your own being

○ To be happy

➤ **This worksheet is available for download at theendofstressbook.com/worksheets.**

Look back over what you checked and consider for a moment how actualizing each of these ways of being would change your day, perhaps even your life. Think of specific situations to which you want to apply each principle, and imagine yourself doing so. Next, imagine realizing the positive result that is inevitable in making this change, and picture it as happening. Place your To-Be List someplace where you will see it, to remind you of how you want to be. You can make a new list whenever you like.

These simple tools add little to your to-do list yet bring empowerment and creative expansion to your day and your life. It's not necessary to use every tool; use whichever tools work for you—but use them. I also encourage you to download this tool and replicate what you have checked in the book on the printed document. Then post it where you will be reminded of your practice. You can make a new list any time you want.

Below is a list of the tools I've presented in this book. It can serve as your daily reminder of practices you want to draw upon to shift from surviving to thriving.

Take the Stress Assessment Again

The last step in pulling it all together is to take the stress assessment again. I invite you to do this to see how your experience of stress has changed since you first did the assessment back in chapter 2. Check off any statements that come close to describing your recent experience of stress. Check off any statements that describe your recent experience of life. Keep your answers current, within the last week or month, and take your time.

Next, refer back to the test you took in chapter 2 at the beginning of this journey. Compare the two tests and highlight what has changed. If you've worked with the tools and processes, a number of items you checked the first time are probably not checked this

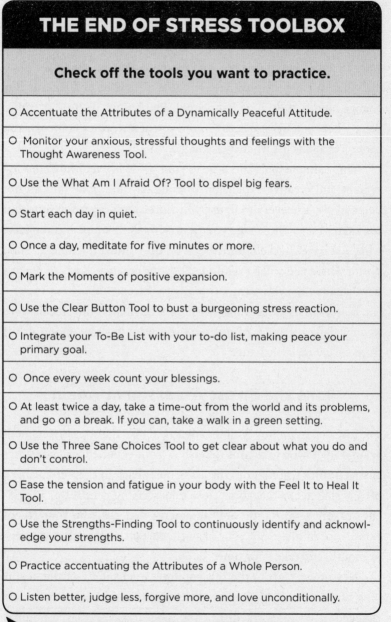

THE END OF STRESS TOOLBOX

Check off the tools you want to practice.

O Accentuate the Attributes of a Dynamically Peaceful Attitude.

O Monitor your anxious, stressful thoughts and feelings with the Thought Awareness Tool.

O Use the What Am I Afraid Of? Tool to dispel big fears.

O Start each day in quiet.

O Once a day, meditate for five minutes or more.

O Mark the Moments of positive expansion.

O Use the Clear Button Tool to bust a burgeoning stress reaction.

O Integrate your To-Be List with your to-do list, making peace your primary goal.

O Once every week count your blessings.

O At least twice a day, take a time-out from the world and its problems, and go on a break. If you can, take a walk in a green setting.

O Use the Three Sane Choices Tool to get clear about what you do and don't control.

O Ease the tension and fatigue in your body with the Feel It to Heal It Tool.

O Use the Strengths-Finding Tool to continuously identify and acknowledge your strengths.

O Practice accentuating the Attributes of a Whole Person.

O Listen better, judge less, forgive more, and love unconditionally.

This worksheet is available for download at theendofstressbook.com/worksheets.

STRESS ASSESSMENT TOOL

O I get less and less pleasure from activities that I used to enjoy.	O I experience fatigue most days and at times become exhausted.
O I have trouble making decisions.	O I'm having difficulty getting to sleep because I can't quiet down, or I'm sleeping more than usual and don't want to get out of bed.
O My memory and concentration are not as good as they used to be.	O I feel less confident about my ability to handle my personal problems.
O Simple things feel burdensome or difficult to accomplish.	O At times I feel overwhelmed and unable to control the important things in my life.
O I have a shorter fuse these days. I'm more impatient, more on edge, and more easily frustrated or annoyed.	O I lose track of little things, such as where I put my keys.
O I experience upsetting emotions such as fear, paranoia, dejection, worry, or pessimism to a greater degree or for prolonged periods.	O I worry over things I can't control.
O I criticize my significant other more, tend to ruminate on the flaws in our relationship, bicker more, and blame my partner for our problems.	O At times, my agitation or frustration can reach the point that I bang on my desk with my fist, throw things, shout, or act out in some other way.
O I've become less social. I find myself wishing that people, including friends and family, would stop bothering me.	O My interest in sex has decreased.
O I eat more to cope with my emotional state, or I have lost my appetite.	O I get sick more often than I think I should, catching colds and flu. I have developed or worry about developing serious health risks.
O My use of alcohol, tobacco, or other substances has increased in part to relieve stress.	O I have tension headaches, gastro-intestinal problems, muscle tension in the back, neck, or jaw, or all of the above.

➤ **This worksheet is available for download at theendofstressbook.com/worksheets.**

time. Using a highlighter pen, mark what you checked on the first test that is not checked on the current test, because it's no longer the issue it was. This indicates the progress you have made in resolving stress-related problems, and there is nothing more encouraging or more motivating than making progress. Taking the stress assessment periodically is an effective way to monitor how you're doing and to motivate you to empower peace even more. You can take the stress assessment anytime by downloading this tool.

Closing

In closing, I want to encourage you to keep going for the Good Life, a life of peace and happiness, free of stress and fear, full of successes achieved through the joy of excelling. The peace, joy, and success you seek are as near as your own thoughts. The formula for neuroplasticity is *Change your mind, change your brain, change your life*. Success is assured if you don't give up. Eventually, significant and lasting results will come . . . if you practice.

I also want to relate a fact of life that I am reminded of every time someone asks me if I ever get stressed. Sometimes, people think that because I've written a book entitled *The End of Stress*, I've ended stress in my life, once and for all. The fact is the end of stress happens or doesn't happen in the present moment—right here, right now—not once and for all. We either end stress by choosing to be at peace the moment a stressor raises its head, or we don't. More often than not, peace is a correction we make when we've allowed a stressor to turn into a mental storm. The quicker we make that correction, the better the day goes.

Just today I was tidying up the house, and the way I was going about it was stressful, making me edgy and tense. I started off fighting with a broken appliance I had to fix and feeling irritated with one of the screws that wouldn't unscrew. It was as if a trickster god was tightening the screw as I was trying to loosen it. Next, I was annoyed at having to unload the dishwasher. As I went about cleaning the rooms, it seemed there was ten times more work than usual. I felt victimized because there was no one to help me, which intensified my bad mood. Then, mercifully, I caught myself in the middle of an unhappy string of self-pitying, resentful thoughts. I have the Thought Awareness Tool to thank for saving me in time. I stopped with the chores for a moment and practiced not believing any of the thoughts my bad mood was thinking. I managed to let go of thinking altogether and gave my mind the chance to quiet down. I made the conscious choice to be present, here and now, and committed to being at peace with whatever I had to do. As I did, these lines came to mind from D. H. Lawrence's poem "We Are Transmitters":

> As we live, we are transmitters of life.
> And when we fail to transmit life, life fails to flow
>   through us.
> . . . .
> Give, and it shall be given unto you
> is still the truth about life.
> . . . .
> It means kindling the life-quality where it was not,
> even if it's only in the whiteness of a washed pocket-
>   handkerchief.[1]

As I recited the lines, my attitude shifted. At that very moment, a cloud blocking the sun passed and the room filled with sunlight. All at once, everything was OK. I felt alive and awake, as bright as the moment. I looked around to see what chores still remained, and set upon them. Work flowed like a dance. As I was raking the last of the leaves in front of the house, a bird flying by caught my eye, and I watched it land in the Japanese maple tree across the street.

It was autumn, and the maple leaves had all turned scarlet red. Some of the leaves were shed, creating a velvet blanket of red on the sidewalk. I looked down the street and noticed that the sycamores were now completely bare. Their branches were dull gray, though the autumn light gave them the look of polished silver in places. From where I stood, the street gradually sloped down to the avenue, and across the avenue was a large field covered in tall green grass. Overhead a falcon, fluttering in midair, scanned the field for prey. Above everything was a pale blue autumn sky. For a moment, I felt completely at peace and at one with the world. As I turned to go back inside the house, I thought that if I hadn't shifted my attitude, I would never have experienced that moment of harmony.

I think we all understand that peace is an inner purpose we work toward every day, and correct to whenever we lose it. You now have the means to empower peace in your life. The test of your progress isn't nirvana. It's in the everyday reality of things becoming better, more harmonious, more joyous, more peaceful and loving. If each day your attitude moves you forward in this way, you are pointed in the right direction.

Stress is fear, and stress free is a form of mastery we can develop that can extinguish psychological fear at the point of inception. No fear, no stress. If you continue to practice being consciously aware of stress reactions when they raise their heads and intervene with a tool or process, your brain will continue to strengthen and expand neural pathways and networks that empower the Good Life. This is the ticket to the health, wealth, and love that this book promised at the beginning. It's all within your reach. This is my sincere wish for you.

As I close this book, I wish you all the grace, dignity, and abundance that peace bestows. This book isn't about you being perfect; it's about progressing toward excelling at life. If stress pulls you into one of its storms, don't become discouraged with yourself. Never quit on yourself and never give up on peace, regardless of the mistakes you make or what is happening around you.

Work for peace, in your heart and in your life. Whenever you fail at peace, take strength in the words of Confucius, who said, "Our greatest glory is not in never falling but in rising every time we fall."[2]

What could define personal strength more than the capacity to transcend stress and fear, and restore the mind to a state of peace and joy? It is one of the great paths to walk, so acknowledge yourself for your willingness to work toward this change in your life.

Anytime you worry that you might regress or that you're not advancing fast enough or that you haven't progressed far enough, correct your state of mind by bringing your attention to the present moment. Simply be right here, right now. Let go of disparaging thoughts and open your mind and heart wide to simply being happy and at peace in this present moment. Remember the words of Thomas Merton that I quoted earlier in the book. Merton said, "All problems are resolved and everything is clear, simply because what matters is clear."[3]

Peace and happiness are what matter and both are restored in the quiet of the present moment. If fear tells you that there are more important things in life than peace, such as money and professional success, remember what this book has documented for you, that an attitude of peace is precisely what recovers and expands the higher brain function that enables you to succeed at every level of life.

In truth, success is inner peace; succeeding is letting go of fear. This one sentence summarizes this entire book. So, be at peace.

Newsletter:
Signup for Don's newletter for the latest breakthroughs in neuroscience and new stress-busting tools.

theendofstressbook.com/signup

Acknowledgments

I first wish to acknowledge my sweetheart, Louise Franklin. She persisted in encouraging me to tackle this writing project and emboldened me to keep going once I started writing. When the project was under way, I was supported by my business partner and close personal friend, Kaarin Alisa. Kaarin helped me conceptualize themes, brainstorm ideas, edit content, and verify facts. I cannot imagine completing this book without Louise or Kaarin.

I want to acknowledge the enormous support this book received from my editors at Beyond Words, Sarah Heilman, Emmalisa Sparrow, and Emily Han, and from managing editor Lindsay Brown. They did a wonderful job of improving the original manuscript, and for that I am grateful.

As always, I want to acknowledge my children, David, Brent, Sam, and Hollan; my sisters, Anne and Susie; and my brother, Paul, for rooting me on.

I want to thank (in no particular order) Bonny Meyer, Larry and Joyce Stupski, Rick Brandon, Cheryl Geoffrion, Andrew Black, Mariah De Leon, Jerry Jampolsky, Diane Cirincione, Jimmy Pete, Mike Johnson, Roger Epstein, Richard Cohn, Dick Buxton, Len Brutoco,

Rinaldo Brutoco, Penelope More, Matthew Mitchell, Greg Sherwood, Patrick Gleeson, David Goewey, Neil Anderson, Jonathan Colton, Marc Verdi, Karen Storsteen, Suzanne Baldwin, Dale Biron, Lorraine Specht, Valerie Henderson, Barbara Deal, Drew Gerber, Michelle Tennant, and everyone else who has assisted me over the years in bringing this work forward.

And finally, I want to acknowledge Cynthia Black, the former president and editor in chief of Beyond Words Publishing. Sadly, Cynthia passed away just as this book was being acquired by Beyond Words. The news of her death came as a shock and saddened me. Cynthia published my first book, *Mystic Cool*, and made me feel so thoroughly welcomed into her illustrious band of authors. I loved working with Cynthia. She was a pioneer in mind, body, and spirit books, and her death diminishes us all.

Appendix:
Healing Type-A

The type-A personality tends to lead a life of extreme stress. Type-A comes out of the landmark research by Meyer Friedman of the University of California, who found that type-A personalities have the highest risk for developing heart disease. The items below represent a somewhat challenging To-Be List that can help anyone who has a type-A personality or suffers from fear-based stress to begin making choices that build a dynamically peaceful attitude. It boils down to a shift from anxiety and stress to peace. Try a few each week, checking them off down the list.

HEALING TYPE-A

Choose one or more of the items below to perform each day until you've done them all. Then repeat the process.

○ Choose the longest line at a store and stand in it, letting your mind go and choosing to be at peace, using the Thirty-Second Time-Out for Peace process.

○ Use a measuring stick other than business to measure your accomplishments; for example, your talents, creative abilities, human qualities, or close relationships.

○ Look out the window for thirty seconds and let your mind go. Watch the wind blow or the sun shine or the rain fall.

○ Devote today to seeing your strengths and positive qualities.

○ Practice forgiving trivial errors.

○ Do one special thing for yourself today.

○ Quietly do good deeds and acts of kindness.

○ Drive home in the slow lane.

○ Practice receiving compliments graciously.

○ Smile more today.

○ Accept that life is unfinished business.

○ Listen to calming music instead of the news on the drive home.

○ Take five minutes today to recall times when you were happy.

○ Practice listening without interrupting.

○ Commit to stop judging yourself for your lack of perfection.

○ Buy a small gift for a friend or family member.

○ Consider the notion that perfection is in the imperfections.

○ Call a good friend you have not talked to in a while.

○ When you feel conflict today, tell yourself, *I am not going to let this person or situation control how I feel*.

○ Look for the best in someone you know.

○ Today, feel more and think less. Become skillful at knowing how you feel by making I feel _____ statements.

➤ **This worksheet is available for download at theendofstressbook.com/worksheets.**

Notes

Foreword

1. Viktor Frankl, *Man's Search for Meaning* (Boston: Beacon, 1992), 75.

Introduction

1. Ask Glenn . . . , "Will computers ever be cleverer than people?," The Science Museum online, http://www.sciencemuseum.org.uk/onlinestuff/snot/will_computers_ever_be_cleverer_than_people.aspx.
2. Janice C. Froehlich, "Opioid Peptides," *Alcohol Health & Research World* 21, no. 2 (1997): 132.
3. G. W. Terman et al., "Intrinsic Mechanisms of Pain Inhibition: Activation by Stress," *Science* 26 (1984): 1270–77.

Chapter 1

1. Norman B. Anderson et al., *Stress in America: Are Teens Adopting Adults' Stress Habits?*, survey commission by the American Psychological Association (February 11, 2014), 3.
2. John Heminway, *Killer Stress: A National Geographic Special*, produced by Stanford University and National Geographic Television (Washington, DC: PBS, premiered September 23, 2008), 00:23:26.
3. Daniel J. Siegel, *Mindsight: The New Science of Personal Transformation* (New York: Bantam, 2009), 8–9.

4. Princeton University, "How Did We Get So Smart? Study Sheds Light On Evolution of the Brain," *ScienceDaily*, May 10, 2001, http://www.sciencedaily.com/releases/2001/05/010510071941.htm.

5. Don Joseph Goewey, *Mystic Cool: A Proven Approach to Transcend Stress, Achieve Optimal Brain Function, and Maximize Your Creative Intelligence* (Hillsboro, OR: Atria/Beyond Words, 2009), 29.

6. Mihaly Csikszentmihalyi, *Flow: The Psychology of Optimal Experience* (New York: Harper Perennial Modern Classics, 2008), 42.

7. Bessel A. van der Kolk, "Memory and the Evolving Psychobiology of Posttraumatic Stress," *Harvard Review of Psychiatry* 1, no. 5 (1994): 263.

8. Joseph LeDoux, *The Emotional Brain: The Mysterious Underpinnings of Emotional Life* (New York: Simon & Schuster, 1996), 167.

9. Wesley E. Sime, *Stress Management: A Review of Principles*, an online series of lectures on stress management, Lecture 1, University of Nebraska, Dept. of Health and Human Performance, 1997, accessed January 2009, http://cehs.unl.edu/stress/resources.html.

10. Harris Interactive, *2013 Work Stress Survey*, on behalf of Everest College, April 9, 2013.

11. Norman B. Anderson et al., *Stress in America: Missing the Health Care Connection*, American Psychological Association (February 7, 2013), 15.

12. Constance Hammen, "Stress and Depression," *Annual Review of Clinical Psychology* 1 (2005): 293–319, http://hammenlab.psych.ucla.edu/pubs/05stressand.pdf.

13. L. E. Kalynchuk et al., "Corticosterone Increases Depression-Like Behavior, with Some Effects on Predator Odor-Induced Defensive Behavior, in Male and Female Rats," *Behavioral Neuroscience* 118, no. 6 (2004): 1365–77. Reported in APA's Science Watch at http://www.apa.org/monitor/jan05/hormones.aspx.

14. *Stress in America*, APA, February 7, 2013, 5.

15. Meghan Neal, "Stress Levels Soar in America by Up to 30% in 30 Years," *New York Daily News*, June 16, 2012, http://www.nydailynews.com/news/national/stress-levels-soar-america-30-30-years-article-1.1096918#ixzz2aNOI4CoA.

16. Timothy A. Judge, Remus Ilies, and Zhen Zhang, "Genetic Influences on Core Self-Evaluations, Job Satisfaction, and Work Stress: A Behavioral Genetics Mediated Model," *Organizational Behavior and Human Decision Processes* 117 (2012): 208–20.

17. University of Notre Dame, "Feeling Stressed by Your Job? Don't Blame Your Employer, Study Shows." *ScienceDaily*, September 14, 2012.

18. R. J. Davidson, J. Kabat-Zinn, et al., "Alterations in Brain and Immune Function Produced by Mindfulness Meditation," *Psychosomatic Medicine* 65 (2003): 564.

19. Elissa S. Epel, Elizabeth H. Blackburn, "Accelerated Telomere Shortening in Response to Life Stress," *Proceedings of the National Academy of Sciences* 101, no. 49 (December 7, 2004): 17312–15.

20. Ibid.

21. Brian Dakss, "Aging: The Stress Factor: Stress, Attitudes Affect DNA, Aging Rates, One Way Or The Other," *CBS News*, August 25, 2005, http://www.cbs news .com/news/aging-the-stress-factor.

22. "How Stress and Mindfulness Affect DNA," Wisdom 2.0 Conference, February 23, 2013.

23. Ibid.

24. Edward Nelson et al., "Longitudinal Associations between Telomere Length, Chronic Stress, and Immune Stance in Cervical Cancer Survivors," *The Journal of Cancer Research* 71, Issue 8, Supplement 1 (April 15, 2011), doi:10.1158/1538-7445.AM2011-1833.

25. Robert M. Sapolsky, *Why Zebras Don't Get Ulcers: An Updated Guide to Stress, Stress Related Diseases, and Coping*, 2nd rev. ed. (New York: W. H. Freeman, 1998), 5.

26. Gregory J. Quirk, René Garcia, and Francisco González-Lima, "Prefrontal Mechanisms in Extinction of Conditioned Fear," *Biological Psychiatry* 60, no. 4 (2006): 337–43, doi:10.1016/j.biopsych.2006.03.010.

Chapter 2

1. Alan Watts, *The Joyous Cosmology: Adventures in the Chemistry of Consciousness* (Novato, CA: New World Library, 2013), 3.

2. C. B. Nemeroff, "The Neurobiology of Depression," *Scientific American* 278, no. 6 (June 1998): 42–9.

3. Joel Schwarz, "Stress Hinders Rats' Decision-Making Abilities," University of Washington, November 18, 2008, http://www.washington.edu/news/2008 /11/18/stress-hinders-rats-decision-making-abilities/.

4. Sime, *Stress Management: A Review of Principles*.

5. S. Qin et al., "Acute Psychological Stress Reduces Working Memory-Related Activity in the Dorsolateral Prefrontal Cortex," *Biological Psychiatry* 66, no. 1 (July 1, 2009): 25–32.

6. S. Vijayraghavan et al., "Inverted-U Dopamine D1 Receptor Actions on Prefrontal Neurons Engaged in Working Memory," *Nature Neuroscience* (February 4, 2007), accelerated online publication.

7. T. Kontogiannis and Z. Kossiavelou, "Stress and Team Performance: Principles and Challenges for Intelligent Decision Aids," *Safety Science* 33, no. 3 (December 1999): 103–28.

8. L. A. Neff and B. R. Karney, "Stress and Reactivity to Daily Relationship Experiences: How Stress Hinders Adaptive Processes in Marriage," *Journal of Personality and Social Psychology* 97 (2009): 435–50.

9. Olga Lechky, "Social Isolation Can Be Major Factor If Patients Are Unable to Deal with Stress," *Canadian Medical Association Journal* 154, no. 4 (1996): 571–72.

10. J. Suls, M. A. Becker, and B. Mullen, "Coronary-Prone Behavior, Social Insecurity and Stress Among College-Aged Adults," *Journal of Human Stress* 7, no. 3 (1981): 27–34.

11. Sapolsky, *Why Zebras Don't Get Ulcers*, 72.

12. Ibid., 347.

13. University of Liverpool, "Stress Hormone Impacts on Alcohol Recovery," *ScienceDaily*, September 23, 2010, http://www.sciencedaily.com/releases/2010 /09/100923104134.htm.

14. Sapolsky, *Why Zebras Don't Get Ulcers*, 62.

15. Ibid., 236.

16. Kalynchuk et al., "Corticosterone Increases," 1365–77.

Chapter 3

1. Harris Interactive, *2013 Work Stress Survey*, April 9, 2013.

2. *Stress in America: Missing the Health Care Connection*, APA 15.

3. Revised from Goewey, *Mystic Cool*, 116.

4. Frankl, *Man's Search for Meaning*, 85.

5. Esther B. Fein, "Book Notes," *New York Times*, November 20, 1991.

6. Frankl, *Man's Search for Meaning*, 116.

7. Ari Ben-Menahem, *Historical Encyclopedia of Natural and Mathematical Sciences*, volume 1 (New York: Springer-Verlag, 2009), 836.

8. Robert L. Leahy, *The Worry Cure: Seven Steps to Stop Worry from Stopping You* (New York: Random House, 2005), 109.

9. Revised from Goewey, *Mystic Cool*, 103–4.

Chapter 5

1. A. M. Graybiel, "The Basal Ganglia and Chunking of Action Repertoires," *Neurobiology of Learning and Memory* 70, nos. 1–2 (1998): 119–36.

2. James Elliot Cabot, *The Works of Ralph Waldo Emerson: A Memoir of Ralph Waldo Emerson* (Cambridge, MA: Riverside Press, 1887), 489.

Chapter 6

1. Anne Lamott, *Operating Instructions: A Journal of My Son's First Year* (New York: Anchor, 1993), 91.

2. William Shakespeare, *The Complete Works* (New York: Harcourt, Brace and World, 1968), from *Macbeth*, 5:5.28, 1216.

3. Ibid., from *Henry VIII*, 3:2.380, 1531.

4. W. B. Yeats, *The Celtic Twilight* (London: A. H. Bullen Publishing, 1902), 136.

5. J. J. Miller, K. Fletcher, and J. Kabat-Zinn, "Effectiveness of a Meditation-Based Stress Reduction Program in the Treatment of Anxiety Disorders," *The American Journal of Psychiatry* 149, no. 7 (July 1, 1992): 936–43.

6. Richard J. Davidson and Antoine Lutz, "Buddha's Brain: Neuroplasticity and Meditation," *IEEE Signal Processing Magazine* 172 (January 2008): 176–79.

7. Thomas Merton, *The Intimate Merton: His Life from His Journals* (New York: HarperOne, 2009), 362.

8. Jill Bolte Taylor, Interview by Robert Krulwich and Jad Abumrad, *Radiolab*, transcript, November 1, 2019, http://reallycoldice.com/2010/11/.

9. Leslie Kaufman, "A Superhighway to Bliss," *New York Times*, May 25, 2008.

10. Modified and expanded from Goewey, *Mystic Cool*, 129–30.

Chapter 7

1. Rudyard Kipling, *Kipling: Poems* (Everyman's Library Pocket Poems) (New York: Knopf, 2007), 172.

2. Bill Utterback, "Athletes Savor Being in 'The Zone'—But No One Has Yet Figured Out How They Can Stay There Forever," *Seattle Times*, March 3, 1991, http://community.seattletimes.nwsource.com/archive/?date=19910303&slug=1269299.

3. Norman Vincent Peale, *The Power of Positive Thinking: 10 Traits for Maximum Results* (New York: Simon & Schuster, 2003), 30.

4. Carlos Castaneda, *Tales of Power* (New York: Washington Square, 1974), 106.

5. Richard S. Lazarus and Susan Folkman, *Stress, Appraisal, and Coping* (New York: Springer, 1984), 19.

6. Eckhart Tolle, *The Power of Now* (Novato, CA: New World Library, 1999), 68.

7. Ed Diener, Eunkook M. Suh, Richard E. Lucas, and Heidi L. Smith, "Subjective Well-Being: Three Decades of Progress," *Psychological Bulletin* 125 (1999): 276–302.

8. Sonya Lyubomirsky, *The How of Happiness: A New Approach to Getting the Life You Want* (New York: Penguin Group, 2007), 22.

9. Sylvain Charron and Etienne Koechlin, "Divided Representation of Concurrent Goals in the Human Frontal Lobes," *Science* 328, no. 5976 (April 2010): 360–63.

10. Eyal Ophir, Clifford Nass, and Anthony D. Wagner, "Cognitive Control in Media Multitaskers," *Proceedings of the National Academy of Sciences* 106, no. 37 (2009): 15583–87.

11. Adam Gorlick, "Media Multitaskers Pay Mental Price, Stanford Study Shows," *Stanford Report*, August 24, 2009, http://news.stanford.edu/news/2009/august24 /multitask-research-study-082409.html.

12. David E. Meyer et al., "Executive Control of Cognitive Processes in Task Switching," *Journal of Experimental Psychology* 27, no. 4 (2001): 763–97.

13. Amanda MacMillan, "12 Reasons to Stop Multitasking," *ABC News*, June 18, 2013, http://abcnews.go.com/Health/Wellness/12-reasons-stop-multitasking /story?id=19422540#2.

14. Erin Hayes, "Slow Down to Get More Done," *ABC News*, May 9, 2008, http:// abcnews.go.com/Technology/story?id=4825616&page=1.

15. Gloria J. Mark and Stephen Voida, "'A Pace Not Dictated by Electrons': An Empirical Study of Work Without Email," presented at the Association for Computing Machinery, May 5, 2012, http://www.ics.uci.edu/~gmark/Home_page /Research_files/CHI%202012.pdf.

16. Revised from Goewey, *Mystic Cool*, 116.

Chapter 8

1. Herbert Benson and Miriam Z. Klipper, *The Relaxation Response* (New York: HarperCollins, 2009), 121.

Chapter 9

1. William James, *William James: Writings, 1878–1899: Psychology, Briefer Course/ The Will to Believe/Talks to Teachers and Students/Essays* (New York: Library of America, 1992), 643.

2. Irena Ilieva, Joseph Boland, and Martha J. Farah, "Objective and Subjective Cognitive Enhancing Effects of Mixed Amphetamine Salts in Healthy People," *Neuropharmacology* (2012), http://dx.doi.org/10.1016/j.neuropharm.2012.07.021.

3. Holly A. White and Priti Shah, "Uninhibited Imaginations: Creativity in Adults with Attention-Deficit/Hyperactivity Disorder," *Personality and Individual Differences* 40 (2006): 1121–31.

4. Denise Mann, "ADHD May Boost Creativity in Adults: Study Shows College Students with ADHD Score Higher on Tests That Measure Creativity," *WebMD*, March 15, 2011, http://www.webmd.com/add-adhd/news/20110315/adhd-may -boost-creativity-in-adults.

5. Peter Galison, "Einstein's Clocks: The Place of Time," *Critical Inquiry* 26, no. 2 (2000): 355–89.

6. Paul D. Kretkowski, "The 15 Percent Solution," *Wired Magazine*, January 23, 1998, http://www.wired.com/techbiz/media/news/1998/01/9858.

7. W. James McNerney Jr., *A Century of Innovation: The 3M Story* (St. Paul, MN: 3M Corporation, 2002), 22.

8. Ibid., 78.

9. "3M Delivers Fourth-Quarter Sales of $7.4 Billion and Earnings of $1.41 per Share; Company Posts Record Full-Year Sales of $29.9 Billion and Earnings of $6.32 per Share," 3M, January 24, 2013, http://media.corporate-ir.net/media _files/IROL/80/80574/4Q_2012_3M_Earnings_Release_4880595.pdf.

10. "3M Performance," 3M, 2013, http://solutions.3m.com/wps/portal/3M/en _US/3M-Company/Information/Profile/Performance/.

11. Kami Goetz, "How 3M Gave Everyone Days Off and Created an Innovation Dynamo," *Fast Company*, February 1, 2011, http://www.fastcodesign.com /1663137/how-3m-gave-everyone-days-off-and-created-an-innovation-dynamo.

12. Agnieszka Wasiak et al., *Lynch: One* (2007), DVD release date August 26, 2008. Absurda/David Lynch, DVD.

13. Karuna Subramaniam et al., "A Brain Mechanism for Facilitation of Insight by Positive Affect," *Journal of Cognitive Neuroscience* 21, no. 3 (March 2009), 415–32.

14. Sarah Zielinski, "5 Ways To Spark Your Creativity," NPR, June 21, 2012, http:// www.npr.org/2012/06/21/155369663/5-ways-to-spark-your-creativity.

15. Ruby T. Nadler, Rahel Rabi, and John Paul Minda, "Better Mood and Better Performance: Learning Rule-Described Categories Is Enhanced by Positive Mood," *Psychological Science* 21, no. 12 (December 2010): 1770–76.

16. Robert Scott Root-Bernstein and Michèle M. Root-Bernstein, *Sparks of Genius: The Thirteen Thinking Tools of the World's Most Creative People* (New York: Houghton Mifflin Harcourt, 1999), 39.

17. Agnes De Mille, *Martha: The Life and Work of Martha Graham—A Biography* (New York: Random House, 1991), 264.

18. John Muir, "The Yellowstone National Park," *The Atlantic Monthly* LXXXI, no. 486 (April 1898): 515–16; modified slightly and reprinted in *Our National Parks* (Cambridge, MA: The Riverside Press, 1901): 56; The Sierra Club, "Quotations from John Muir: selected by Harold Wood," http://www.sierraclub.org/john_muir _exhibit/writings/favorite_quotations.aspx.

19. R. Sperry, "Hemisphere Deconnection and Unity in Consciousness," *American Psychologist* 23 (1968): 723–33.

20. Harnam Singh and Michael W. O'Boyle, "Interhemispheric Interaction During Global-Local Processing in Mathematically Gifted Adolescents, Average-Ability Youth, and College Students," *Neuropsychology* 18, no. 2 (April 2004): 371–77.

21. Jan Ehrenwald, *Anatomy of Genius: Split Brains and Global Minds* (New York: Human Sciences Press, 1984), 16.

22. Robert Sperry, "Some Effects of Disconnecting the Cerebral Hemispheres," Nobel Media, December 23, 2013, http://www.nobelprize.org/nobel_prizes/medicine/laureates/1981/sperry-lecture_en.html?print=1.

23. Marjorie Lamberti, *The Politics of Education: Teachers and School Reform in Weimar Germany* (New York: Berghahn Books, 2004), 28, quoting Wilhelm Reese.

24. Cheryl Lavin, "Thinking Is the Enemy of Creativity. It's Self-Conscious . . . ," *Chicago Tribune*, November 16, 1997.

25. John D. Norton, "Goodies," Department of History and Philosophy of Science and Center for Philosophy of Science, University of Pittsburgh, updated May 6, 2013, http://www.pitt.edu/~jdnorton/Goodies.

26. John Kounios et al., "The Origins of Insight in Resting-State Brain Activity," *Neuropsychologia* 46 (2008): 282.

27. Jonah Lehrer, *Imagine: How Creativity Works* (New York: Houghton Mifflin Harcourt, 2012), 16.

28. "Brain Waves and Meditation," *ScienceDaily*, March 31, 2010, http://www.sciencedaily.com/releases/2010/03/100319210631.htm.

29. *Lee Ufan: Marking Infinity*, Guggenheim Museum, Sackler Center for Art Education, Family Activity Guide, September 2011.

30. Arthur Herman, *How the Scots Invented the Modern World: The True Story of How Western Europe's Poorest Nation Created Our World and Everything in It* (New York: Random House, 2007), 321.

31. "Basic Rest and Activity Cycles," Polyphasic Society, http://www.polyphasicsociety.com/polyphasic-sleep/science/brac/.

32. Ibid.

33. K. Anders Ericsson, Ralf Krampe, and Clemens Tesch-Romer, "The Role of Deliberate Practice in the Acquisition of Expert Performance," *Psychological Review* 100, no. 3 (1993): 363–406.

34. Michelle W. Voss et al., "Plasticity of Brain Networks in a Randomized Intervention Trial of Exercise Training in Older Adults," *Frontiers in Aging Neuroscience* 2, no. 32 (2010), 1.

35. "A Walk a Day Keeps the Doctor at Bay," University of Essex, May 2, 2010, http://www.essex.ac.uk/news/event.aspx?e_id=1588.

36. W. Sommer et al., "How about Lunch? Consequences of the Meal Context on Cognition and Emotion," *PLoS ONE* 8, no. 7 (2013): e70314, doi:10.1371/journal.pone.0070314.

37. Benjamin Baird et al., "Inspired by Distraction: Mind Wandering Facilitates Creative Incubation," *Psychological Science* (August 31, 2012), 1117–22, doi: 0956797612446024.

38. Lehrer, *Imagine*, 32–33.

39. R. A. Emmons and M. E. McCullough, "Counting Blessings Versus Burdens: An Experimental Investigation of Gratitude and Subjective Well-Being in Daily Life," *Journal of Personality and Social Psychology* 84, no. 2 (2003): 377–89, doi: 10.1037/0022-3514.84.2.377.

40. Annette Bolte, Thomas Goschke, and Julius Kuhl, "Emotion and Intuition: Effects of Positive and Negative Mood on Implicit Judgments of Semantic Coherence," *Psychological Science* 14 (2003): 416–22.

41. "Count Your Blessings," Health and Happiness, *Time*, 2006, http://xontent.time.com/time/specials/2007/article/0,28804,1631176_1630611_1630512,00.html.

42. A. Goldstein et al., "Unilateral Muscle Contractions Enhance Creative Thinking," *Psychonomic Bulletin & Review* 17, no. 6 (December 2010): 895–99.

43. R. E. Propper et al., "Getting a Grip on Memory: Unilateral Hand Clenching Alters Episodic Recall," *PLoS ONE* 8 (April 24, 2013): e62474.

44. William W. Maddux and Adam D. Galinsky, "Cultural Borders and Mental Barriers: The Relationship between Living Abroad and Creativity," *Journal of Personality and Social Psychology* 96, no. 5 (May 2009): 1047–61.

45. Marily Oppezzo and Daniel L. Schwartz, "Give Your Ideas Some Legs: The Positive Effect of Walking on Creative Thinking," *Journal of Experimental Psychology: Learning, Memory, and Cognition* 4, no. 4 (July 2014): 1142–1152.

45. University of California, Berkeley, "Remote Associates Test," last updated January 11, 2011, http://socrates.berkeley.edu/~kihlstrm/RATest.htm.

Chapter 10

1. Eduardo Dias-Ferreira et al., "Chronic Stress Causes Frontostriatal Reorganization and Affects Decision-Making," *Science* 325, no. 5940 (July 31, 2009): 621–25.

2. Natalie Angier, "Brain Is a Co-Conspirator in a Vicious Stress Loop," *New York Times*, August 18, 2009.

3. Ellen Galinsky et al., *Overwork in America: When the Way We Work Becomes Too Much* (Families and Work Institute, 2005), 7.

4. "PGi Finds 82% of Employees Choose to Stay Connected to the Office While on Vacation," PR Newswire, August 26, 2013, http://www.prnewswire.com/news-releases/pgi-finds-82-of-employees-choose-to-stay-connected-to-the-office-while-on-vacation-221148391.html.

5. Stephanie Rosenbloom, "Please Don't Make Me Go on Vacation," *New York Times*, August 10, 2006.

Chapter 11

1. Sigmund Freud, *Civilization and Its Discontents* (New York: Norton, 2005), 123–24.

2. Brené Brown, *I Thought It Was Just Me (But It Isn't): Making the Journey from "What Will People Think?" to "I Am Enough,"* (New York: Gotham Books, 2007), Kindle edition, Kindle location: 638–39.

3. Holly VanScoy, "Shame: The Quintessential Emotion," *PsychCentral*, January 30, 2013, http://psychcentral.com/lib/shame-the-quintessential-emotion/000730.

4. Carl R. Rogers, *A Way of Being* (New York: Houghton Mifflin Harcourt, 1995), 123–28.

5. Amy Maxmen, "Secret Shame: Do You Fear What Others Think of You? How Shame Can Hurt Your Health," *Psychology Today*, October 26, 2007, http://www.psychologytoday.com/articles/200710/secret-shame.

6. S. Dickerson, T. Gruenewald, and M. Kemeny, "Shame, Physiology, and Health," *Journal of Personality* 72, no. 6 (December 2004): 1191–1210.

7. Siegel, *Mindsight: The New Science of Personal Transformation*, 3.

8. Martin Seligman, *Learned Optimism: How to Change Your Mind and Your Life* (New York: Free Press, 1990), 129–30.

9. Suzanne Retzinger, "Identifying Shame and Anger in Discourse," *American Behavioral Scientist* 38, no. 8 (August 1995): 104–13.

10. Donald L. Nathanson, *Shame and Pride: Affect, Sex, and the Birth of the Self* (New York: W. W. Norton & Company, 1994), 313–14.

11. Thomas M. Scheff and Suzanne M. Retzinger, "Shame, Anger and the Social Bond: A Theory of Sexual Offenders and Treatment," *Electronic Journal of Sociology* 1 (September 1997): 2.

12. Allan N. Schore, *Affect Dysregulation and Disorders of the Self* (New York: Norton, 2008), 160.

13. Brian Thorne and Pete Sanders, *Carl Rogers* (Thousand Oaks, CA: SAGE Publications, 2012), 28.

14. "Albert Ellis—On Guilt and Shame—RARE 1960 recording, part 2," uploaded by ProfessorMystic to YouTube, June 4, 2009, http://www.youtube.com/watch?v=tuNWeI_l0F4.

15. Ibid.

16. Herbert Arthur Otto, *A Guide to Developing Your Potential* (North Hollywood, CA: Wilshire Book Co., 1977), 172.

17. Marcus Buckingham and Donald O. Clifton, *Now, Discover Your Strengths* (New York: Free Press, 2001), 6–8.

18. Brené Brown, "Listening to Shame," TED, March 2012, http://www.ted.com/talks/brene_brown_listening_to_shame.html.

19. Carl Rogers, *On Becoming a Person: A Therapist's View of Psychotherapy* (New York: Houghton Mifflin Harcourt, 2012), 183–91.

20. Alan W. Watts, *Psychotherapy East and West* (New York: Vintage, 1975), 28.

21. Joan M. Cook, Tatyana Biyanova, and James C. Coyne, "Influential Psychotherapy Figures, Authors, and Books: An Internet Survey of Over 2,000," *Psychotherapy: Theory, Research, Practice, Training* 46, no. 1 (March 2009): 42–51.

22. Rogers, *On Becoming a Person*, 194.

23. Daniel Siegel, *The Mindful Brain: Reflection and Attunement in the Cultivation of Well-Being* (New York: Norton, 2007), 41–44.

Chapter 12

1. Dan Buettner, *The Blue Zones: 9 Lessons for Living Longer From the People Who've Lived the Longest*, second ed., (National Geographic Society, 2012), Kindle edition, 227–29.

2. John G. Bruhn and Stewart Wolf, *The Roseto Story* (Norman, OK: University of Oklahoma Press, 1979), 41.

3. John G. Bruhn and Stewart Wolf, *The Power of Clan: The Influence of Human Relationships on Heart Disease* (New Brunswick, NJ: Transaction Publishers, 1998), 10.

4. Clarke Johnson, "The Roseto Effect, Hominid Evolution, Dental Anthropology, and Human Variation," University of Illinois at Chicago, Course Notes 14.2, 1–6, http://www.uic.edu/classes/osci/osci590/14_2%20The%20Roseto%20Effect.htm.

5. Julianne Holt-Lunstad, Timothy B. Smith, and J. Bradley Layton, "Social Relationships and Mortality Risk: A Meta-analytic Review," *PLoS Med* 7, no. 7 (July 27, 2010): e1000316, doi:10.1371/journal.pmed.1000316.

6. Ibid.

7. Jeanna Bryner, "Kids to Parents: Leave the Stress at Work," Associated Press, January 23, 2007.

8. Public Relations Staff, "APA Stress Survey: Children Are More Stressed than Parents Realize," American Psychological Association, November 23, 2009, http://www.apapracticecentral.org/update/2009/11-23/stress-survey.aspx.

9. Daniel Goleman, "Friends for Life: An Emerging Biology of Emotional Healing," *New York Times*, October 10, 2006.

10. Ker Than, "Scientists Say Everyone Can Read Minds," *Live-Science*, April 27, 2006, http://www.livescience.com/health/050427_mind_readers.html.

11. Marco Iacoboni, *Mirroring People: The New Science of How We Connect with Others* (New York: Farrar, Straus and Giroux, 2009), 119.

12. Deborah J. Laible, Gustavo Carlo, and Scott C. Roesch, "Pathways to Self-Esteem in Late Adolescence: The Role of Parent and Peer Attachment, Empathy, and Social Behaviors," *Journal of Adolescence* 27, no. 6 (December 2004): 703–16.

13. Rogers, *A Way of Being*, 137.

14. Ibid., 137–40.

15. Michele W. Atkins, "Course: The Empathic Leader," PowerPoint presentation, Union University, 2001, slide 9.

Chapter 13

1. R. B. Michael, M. Garry, and I. Kirsch, "Suggestion, Cognition, and Behavior," *Current Directions in Psychological Science* 21, no. 3 (2012): 151–56.

2. "The Power of Suggestion: What We Expect Influences Our Behavior, for Better or Worse," News, Association for Psychological Science, June 6, 2012, http://www .psychologicalscience.org/index.php/news/releases/the-power-of-suggestion -what-we-expect-influences-our-behavior-for-better-or-worse.html.

3. Robert Pagliarini, "Meet Bruce Lee, Personal Growth Guru," CBS/MoneyWatch, August 27, 2012, http://www.cbsnews.com/news/meet-bruce-lee-personal -growth-guru/.

4. Henry K. Beecher, "Relationship of Significance of Wound to Pain Experienced," *JAMA* 161, no. 17 (1956) 1609–13, doi:10.1001/jama.1956.02970170005002.

5. Sophie Parker et al., "A Sham Drug Improves a Demanding Prospective Memory Task," *Memory* 19, no. 6 (August 2011): 606–12.

6. Ben Colagiuri, Evan J. Livesey, and Justin A. Harris, "Can Expectancies Produce Placebo Effects for Implicit Learning?" *Psychonomic Bulletin Review* 18 (2011): 399–405, doi:10.3758/s13423-010-0041-1.

7. M. McClung and D. Collins, "'Because I Know It Will!': Placebo Effects of an Ergogenic Aid on Athletic Performance," *Journal of Sport & Exercise Psychology* 29, no. 3 (2007): 382–94.

8. Ellen J. Langer, *Counterclockwise: Mindful Health and the Power of Possibility* (New York: Random House, 2009), 5–12.

9. Alia J. Crum and Ellen J. Langer, "Mind-Set Matters: Exercise and the Placebo Effect," *Psychological Science* 18, no. 2 (2007): 165–71.

10. "Believing Is Seeing: How Mindset Can Improve Vision," Association for Psychological Science, April 9, 2010, http://www.psychologicalscience.org/media /releases/2010/langer.cfm.

11. Thomas Merton, *The Intimate Merton: His Life from His Journals*, ed. Patrick Hart and Jonathan Montaldo (San Francisco: HarperSanFrancisco, 1996), 161.

12. Lisa Liddane, "The Power of Suggestion: Hypnosis," *Orange County Register*, August 20, 2006.

Closing

1. D. H. Lawrence, "We Are Transmitters," *Selected Poems* (New York: Viking, 1959), 105.

2. Confucius, "Quotes by Confucius," Quotations Book, accessed April 23, 2014, http://quotationsbook.com/quotes/author/1644/confucius/all/.

3. Merton, *The Intimate Merton: His Life from His Journals*, 362.

THE END OF STRESS

GUIDED PROCESSES AUDIO DOWNLOAD

http://www.beyondword.com/endofstress

Do not listen to these recordings while operating a motor vehicle or any machinery.

Running time approximately 62 minutes / ℗ & © by Don Joseph Goewey.